You are Not Alone

Life After a Breast Cancer Diagnosis

Andrea Schneider

authorHOUSE®

AuthorHouse™
1663 Liberty Drive
Bloomington, IN 47403
www.authorhouse.com
Phone: 1-800-839-8640

First published by AuthorHouse 7/30/2010

ISBN: 978-1-4520-3823-0 (e)
ISBN: 978-1-4520-3822-3 (sc)
ISBN: 978-1-4520-3821-6 (hc)

Printed in the United States of America
Bloomington, Indiana

This book is printed on acid-free paper.

Cover photo by Nancee E. Lewis.

Acknowledgments

I am so grateful to my family for allowing me the time to write this book and for helping me through my most difficult moments in life. A special thank you to my mom and daughter, Gabby, for taking care of me, being sources of strength, and for looking at my breasts when I didn't have the courage to do so. Thanks also to my young son, Andrew, who wouldn't allow me to feel sorry for myself. I acknowledge all of my friends and family who gave me support and encouragement over the last few years. You never made me feel different because I had cancer, and I appreciate you all. Thank you to my remarkable medical staff, especially Dr. S. who helped me to feel whole and complete.

Finally, I'd like to thank my knowledgeable contributor, Dr. Barry Handler; my tremendous editor, Suzan Tusson; my amazing photographer, Nancee Lewis; and the wonderful Neysa Whiteman, M.D., Board Certified FACOG (Fellow of the American College of Obstetrics and Gynecology) for her valuable input and corrections.

Foreward

When you are diagnosed with cancer you are faced with decisions to make about your treatment that you may be completely unprepared to make. These are choices that must be made in a timely fashion that in some instances can never be undone. You are suddenly in a maelstrom of doctor appointments with long waits in the waiting room, tests that are sometimes painful, and results in medical jargon that you do not understand.

Despite support from family and friends, you are overwhelmed, fearful of the "worse case scenarios" you have read about on the internet, and probably not sleeping much at all. You wish that one physician who you trust will tell you exactly what to do and make all of your appointments for you. But, more often than not, there will be several physicians with different opinions and you will have to make some of these difficult life changing decisions on your own. Where do you start?

Andrea has shared her own journey down this path and done many hours of research. Reading her book will give you the basic information that you need to speak to your physician intelligently and understand the ramifications of the choices that you may be asked to make.

Neysa Whiteman, M.D.-Board Certified FACOG (Fellow of the American College of Obstetrics and Gynecology)

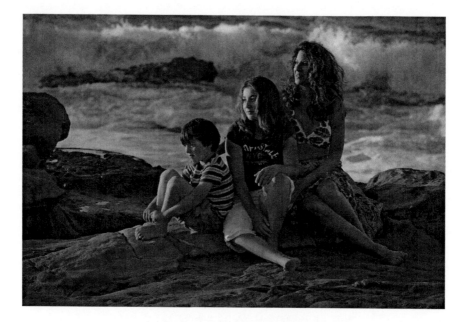

YOU ARE NOT ALONE:
LIFE AFTER A BREAST CANCER DIAGNOSIS
BY ANDREA SCHNEIDER, ESQ.
WITH CONTRIBUTIONS BY BARRY HANDLER, MD.

Table of Contents

YOU ARE NOT ALONE: LIFE AFTER A BREAST CANCER DIAGNOSIS
BY ANDREA SCHNEIDER, ESQ.
WITH CONTRIBUTIONS BY BARRY HANDLER, MD.

INTRODUCTION

Reasons for writing this book:

- **To share my experiences and knowledge with other women.**
- **To let women know they are not alone.**
- **To empower women so they can make decisions which are right for them.**
- **To give my readers the confidence, hope, inspiration, and knowledge they will need to make it through this challenging time.**
- **To re-iterate that early detection saves lives. Medical experts rarely mention that early detection saves breasts. In our society, women should not die of breast cancer. It is our responsibility to stay on top of screening and self-examination. Don't watch and wait! What are you waiting for? For the cancer to spread into your body? Your breasts and, most certainly, your life are at stake.**
- **To vent.**
- **To reach out to as many women as I can, though if I only help one woman then it was worth writing.**

This book is primarily for women who have been diagnosed with breast cancer, yet it can also benefit women at risk of being diagnosed with breast cancer, which is pretty much any woman. If you become the one in eight women who gets breast cancer, realize you are not alone, and that most breast cancer is treatable. Please read my book with care, take notes if you like, write in the margins and be sure to ask your doctor all of your questions.

This book is not meant to scare you, but rather to arm you with the knowledge you will need to get through the breast cancer experience. This book will not provide every answer but, hopefully, you will find it thought provoking. If something in the book particularly interests or concerns you, I encourage you to do your own research.

If you are one of the fortunate women who have not been diagnosed with breast cancer, I recommend you read this book anyway for future reference for yourself or someone you know who may get breast cancer. Be aware, however, that some of the content of this book may not be clear to you if you have not been diagnosed with breast cancer.

1. ME

MY HISTORY:

Born in 1964, I grew up in a Chicago suburb called Des Plaines. Although I didn't know any attorneys or anyone from California, somehow I knew that I would become an attorney and live in California. I felt certain I would go to college even though my parents had no money saved for my education. While researching colleges, my brother's friend's mother offered to help. She brought me to Lake Forest College (LFC) for an interview. Her act of kindness changed the direction of my life. LFC is an outstanding private school with only about 1100 students. LFC provided me scholarships, a work study program, financial aid, and an exceptional education.

During my senior year, I interned in the Antitrust Department of the Attorney General's Office. I thought I'd learn about the legal profession and decide if I really wanted to become an attorney. On my first day the head attorney said, "Here is your desk, all you need to do is sit here and look pretty," in 1986 that was acceptable language and behavior. If anything, the internship encouraged me not to go to law school.

I graduated Cum Laude from Lake Forest College in May of 1986 with a major in Economics. After graduation I spent a year at Tel Aviv University in Israel studying Middle Eastern Studies in their graduate program.

After that, I moved to Arizona to be with my family. I sold health insurance and tried some multi-level marketing programs. After a few years, I decided that if I was ever going to go to law school, I better just do it. I enrolled at California Western School of Law in San Diego, California where I received an academic scholarship for my first year. I attended law school from 1989-1992.

Late 1991/Early 1992

I first noticed a lump in my breast around the end of 1991 or early 1992 at 27 years old. My ob-gyn said, "Cut down on caffeine and come back in a few months." I later returned, and she thought everything felt fine. I didn't have insurance at the time so I didn't pursue this any further. Somewhere in the back of my head I remember thinking I would have breast cancer some day. I hoped I was wrong. A woman's intuition rarely is.

After law school, while studying for the California bar exam, I drank up to seven cups of coffee a day and also ate chocolate covered Expresso beans. I didn't even like coffee, but I needed the caffeine to stay awake, read, and study. After the bar exam I gave up coffee and tried to limit my caffeine intake, yet I never stopped eating a small amount of milk chocolate every day.

I took the bar exam at the end of July 1992 but didn't get results until the weekend of Thanksgiving. Thankfully I passed the test the first time, and I was sworn into the California bar on December 1, 1992. I began my first job as an attorney on December 3, 1992. The Alternate Public Defender's Office hired me as an independent contractor to assist an older, accomplished attorney with a murder case in which the client faced the death penalty. I thought this case would take six months, but it actually took 2.5 years.

While finishing up this case, I prepared to open my own office. In the beginning of 1995, I established my law office with a focus on criminal defense. While working on John's trial I met a reporter, Paul, who was covering it. I later ran into Paul, and he hired me to help him with some contracts for his business. After finishing my work for Paul, we began dating. Fourteen years later we are still together and now have two children, Gabby and Andrew. We never know who we will meet or when we will meet them. If it weren't for John and his nasty case, I may never have met Paul and my life would have been totally different.

October of 1996

I had my daughter, Gabriela at nearly 32 years old. I breastfed her for about four or five weeks; she wasn't that into it and neither was I. I found it to be hard work. Bottle feeding seemed so much easier for us. Being self-employed, I had no maternity leave and didn't take any time off after having Gabby. Even though I had a profession, being a mom came first. Thus, I worked around Gabby's schedule.

Late 1998

I felt a lump in my right breast. I was referred to a surgeon, Dr. L. She was going to do a needle biopsy but confirmed my idea that a needle biopsy is not always accurate. False readings are possible. Due to my age, 34, my breasts were very dense (not much fat). She shared that a mammogram would probably not show anything. I don't recall if I had a mammogram, an ultrasound, or neither of these tests. I chose to have the lump surgically removed via a biopsy. In late December of 1998, I had the lump taken out and it was fine. A year or two later I felt something in that same spot again. Over the years Dr. L performed a few biopsies in that same area because something hard kept growing there.

POINTS FROM DR. BARRY:

- **Mammograms look at breast density and are most useful when a woman is over 40. Her breasts are less dense then and contain more fat.**
- **A tumor is denser than fatty tissue so it shows up better when being compared to fatty tissue.**
- **An ultrasound shoots sound waves into the tissue. The waves are reflected back and indicate how far away the lump is, and if it is solid or fluid.**

3

- **Mammograms and ultrasounds can not detect atypical CELLS.**
- **A biopsy can detect atypical cells.**

2002

I had a lump surgically removed via a biopsy and this time the medical team determined that my tissue had "atypical cells." They did not recommend any special treatment, diet, or anything else. I began getting mammograms and sometimes had an ultrasound every year. Nothing suspicious showed up during these tests. I continued my self-exams on an often too frequent basis. I was hyper-vigilent about self exams and getting mammograms.

Late 2003/early 2004

I felt something again in the same area of previous biopsies, near the armpit area of my right breast. Dr. L thought it was probably scar tissue yet I chose to have it surgically removed on February 16, 2004. I didn't know at the time that I was a few days pregnant. All went well with my biopsy.

I turned 40 in September and gave birth to my son, Andrew, on November 11, 2004. Both the pregnancy and the delivery progressed smoothly, and we were both healthy. None of my doctors ever discussed the effect pregnancy and nursing might have with my breast cancer risks. In the hospital the lactation people pushed nursing and were more concerned about my breastfeeding than how I might be feeling.

POINTS FROM DR. BARRY:

- **Pregnancy does not increase the risk of getting breast cancer.**
- **Breastfeeding may decrease the risk of getting breast cancer.**

Andrew nursed right away. He loved it, and it worked for me. I now had my own mortgage business and did most of my work from home. I had a very flexible schedule. During the first week of nursing, my breast became red, swollen, and sore. I had a breast infection/mastitis. My doctor prescribed antibiotics. I took them and felt fine a few days later. Andrew had taken to the nursing so much I joked that I would have to cut him off my boob before he went to college so he wouldn't get teased by his roommates. I also remembered hearing that breastfeeding decreases a woman's risk of getting breast cancer which also encouraged me along.

I later found out from my insurance plan that they wouldn't allow me to get a mammogram while still breastfeeding and not until I had ceased nursing for six months. But, as you will see somehow they managed to give me a mammogram about a month after I stopped breastfeeding, which was after I got diagnosed with breast cancer. I also didn't realize that while nursing I wouldn't get my period. I appreciated this nice bonus for 18 months. I later learned that not being on my menstrual cycle while breastfeeding may help decrease the risk of getting breast cancer. As I will discuss later, it appears the less ovulation cycles you have in your lifetime, actually lower your risk of getting breast cancer.

Mid 2005

I felt something solid again in my right breast where I had previous biopsies. I called my medical provider to find out what to do. They told me that my prior breast surgeon, Dr. L had moved out of state. I played phone tag with her nurse, Cynthia, to refer me to another surgeon. I spoke to several people at my HMO/insurance plan, and each one told me something different about whether I could get a mammogram while still nursing or how long I would have to wait for one after breastfeeding.

December of 2005

I went to see the Surgeon, Dr. X. Based on the number of biopsies I had previously, she felt it was probably scar tissue that we were feeling. I had an ultrasound, and it did not show anything abnormal.

5

I had a needle biopsy and it showed no cancer. We decided to wait a few months and then re-examine the area.

During this waiting period my sister-in-law Pauline highly recommended I try an acupuncturist. The one she referred me to had successfully treated my mother for Bells Palsy. The acupuncturist is an interesting Asian woman who caressed my hand, felt my finger nail and then instinctively, without me telling her where my lump was, touched the exact spot of the lump. This Spiritual woman astonished me. I visited her 10 times to get rid of the lump and increase my energy. She told me I didn't have breast cancer because if I did she would "taste it." With her English not being so great, I'm still not sure if the acupuncturist meant she would "taste it" through some intuitive way or that my skin would somehow feel funny to her touch. I never clarified this with her.

Somehow, during the course of my treatment with the acupuncturist, the substantial scar from my previous biopsies pretty much disappeared, and the lump seemed smaller to me, or maybe gone. I was pretty impressed. I felt certain I didn't have breast cancer. I returned to Dr. X to tell her about my success with the acupuncturist. I expected her to say I didn't need a biopsy since the scar had pretty much disappeared, and I didn't feel the lump as much as before. But she said that the lump had become more pronounced than before.

I continued nursing my son Andrew, so they wouldn't give me a mammogram until six months after I finished breastfeeding. I felt certain I didn't have breast cancer but wanted to confirm it.

I breastfed Andrew for almost 18 months, until May 2nd, and then switched him to the left breast so I could have the lump removed from my right breast on May 4th, 2006. Dr. X told me that I needed to stop breastfeeding before the biopsy. I recently learned that you don't necessarily have to stop breast feeding before a biopsy.

POINTS FROM DR. BARRY:

- **Technically you can operate on a breast that has been breastfeeding.**
- **But, operating on a lactating breast can increase the risk of infections and may make it harder to heal.**

May 4, 2006

Dr. X felt my breast and said it seemed the same as the last time she checked it. She asked if I still wanted to have the lump surgically removed or if I'd rather wait and watch it some more. I decided to have the lump taken out and biopsied. She anesthetized the area and removed the lump in her office. She informed me the whole time about what she was doing. Her sharing too much information about what she was feeling and how deep she was going made me a bit nauseous. We also talked about my upcoming trip to Italy and some of her travels. Dr. X used some kind of cauterizing stick during the surgery so I didn't bleed much. The procedure took about half an hour and, overall, I found it tolerable. Paul drove me home about an hour afterward and I felt okay, except for a stiff arm, probably from the awkward position I had it in during the procedure.

MY DIAGNOSIS

May 10, 2006

While driving home from the store with Andrew and my then nine year old daughter, Gabby, I received a call from Dr. X. She was speaking fast and said, "I have good and bad news. The good news is you have very early, stage 0, breast cancer called DCIS-*ductal carcinoma in situ*, a single cell cancer that is not invasive cancer but could become invasive cancer if left untreated. The bad news, it is a cancer or some deem it pre-cancer." She had found 3 mm (a little smaller than a pencil eraser) of high grade DCIS but it was only .5 mm from a margin (very close to a margin or edge). Thus, she needed to go in and take more out to see if we could get a clean margin.

She may have thought she had some good news to share, yet I didn't think any kind of cancer could be positive. Also, it is not a good idea to tell a patient he/she has cancer over the phone, especially when one is driving.

She wanted me to have surgery in two days. She said if she went in, took out more tissue, and they found no more cancer, then I would probably be done. Alternatively, if they found more cancer then I would need to consult with an oncologist, a radiation therapist, and have a mammogram.

When Dr. X phoned, I pulled over to the side of the road, wrote down what she said, asked some questions, hung up, and burst out crying. No one wants to hear the word "carcinoma." I finally felt more myself and could fully move my arm when I received news that I needed to be cut again. From the side of the road, I called Paul to share the news. He told me not to over-react and cleared his schedule for my upcoming surgery. I next phoned my mom in Chicago where she was visiting my brother and family. She cut her trip short and came home the next day to provide me with moral support and to help with the kids.

May 12, 2006

I returned to the hospital. This time I had general anesthesia. They put me to sleep so that Dr. X could go deeper and take out more tissue than she had taken out in the biopsy eight days before. The news that she wanted the surgery scheduled so quickly, along with my need to be put under in a hospital, rather than an outpatient setting as before, felt unsettling. I realized my situation could be more serious than she was telling me.

One of my fears is not waking up from anesthesia. I always ask the doctor to give me just enough so I will sleep through the procedure but I want to wake up right after it. Paul drove me to the hospital. While there they administered an IV as I talked to the anesthesiologist. Soon I was in a deep sleep. I went home a few hours after the biopsy. Again my arm seemed stiff for a few days, and I couldn't drive for a few days. Other than the mental anxiety, I felt pretty good.

May 19, 2006

Dr. X called to tell me they discovered more high grade DCIS in a deeper area than the original cancer site. My diagnosis had now become *multi focal Ductal Carcinoma in Situ*, meaning that the DCIS was found in more than one place. The good news was that no invasive cancer was found. The two separate cancer sites were separated by about 3 to 4 centimeters (about an inch to an inch and a half). The second spot of DCIS was 1.6 millimeters (about half of a pencil eraser) yet again was close to a margin. Dr. X had re-excised (taken out) 5 centimeters of my breast tissue, about 2 inches. I didn't even realize that much was taken out in the second surgery until later converting centimeters to inches.

They located a very small spot of cancer in the 2 inch sample of tissue. As Dr. X said, "a few stupid cells were found near the surgical margin." She mentioned that if she took out more tissue, she could possibly find more cancer cells. It was also possible that the two found spots were all I had. I asked Dr. X if my recent breastfeeding had been taken into account, and she said that breastfeeding does not change cells. She also shared that neither an ultrasound nor a mammogram could detect these cancer cells. Either way the lump had been removed. She encouraged me to take action because DCIS could become an invasive cancer. Dr. X said, "You should call the oncologist in three days, and the radiation therapy people will call you."

DCIS (ductal carcinoma in situ) means that the cancer cells were in my ducts and thought to be stationary rather than spreading, thus becoming invasive. I had no symptoms to indicate anything was wrong with me other than a lump which kept reoccurring. I do not believe women with DCIS have any symptoms. Strangely enough, according to Dr. X, the lump I kept feeling was actually fine. When Dr. X performed the first biopsy, she probed a little deeper, noticed something grainy, and took it out. They found the DCIS in the deeper area. I felt grateful to know about the DCIS yet also sad to learn about it at the same time. What would I do now?

Dr. X told me she believed many women have dormant DCIS and that it is good and bad when it is discovered. You almost don't want to find it. The reality is that if cancer is present, it is probably best to find out. Yet learning you have cancer is difficult because no one wants to have it, on any level. A cancer diagnosis will put your life in a tailspin.

May of 2006

I tried to be objective and take myself out of the equation. I decided to approach breast cancer as a research project or as a problem a client or friend needed help to find the best solution for. My training as an attorney definitely helped me with this.

With my new cancer diagnosis of *multi focal Ductal Carcinoma in Situ*, I began doing a lot of research on the internet. The recommended treatment choices shocked me. With an early stage breast cancer diagnosis I thought I would either take a pill for a few weeks and/or they would clean out my ducts. Instead many internet sites I looked at indicated that for multi focal (found in more than one place in the duct), DCIS (ductal carcinoma *in situ*) meaning cancer found in the duct yet contained in that area, the choices were radiation to the site followed by Tamoxifen and other drugs after that; or a mastectomy.

How could the choices be so extreme for such early stage breast cancer? DCIS is considered stage 0 cancer! Some sites even refer to DCIS as pre-cancer. I told Paul, what I read about on the internet and shared my feelings on what I'd like to do next. He thought that I was over-reacting and needed to wait and talk to the oncologist. When you do research on the internet, be careful that you are looking at legitimate sites and not sites that are trying to sell you something. Always consider your source.

I found the site, http://www.4woman.gov/faq/earlybc.htm, by The National Women's Health Information Center to be very helpful. The 10 page article entitled "Early Stage Breast Cancer: A Patient and Doctor Dialogue" defined terminology and answered a lot of my questions. It discussed treatment options for early stage breast cancer and offered pros and cons for each choice. It also listed the survival rates for each treatment option. It seemed to me that this site leaned more toward radiation possibly combined with Tamoxifen as the suggested treatment for most early stage breast cancer. The article also stated, "if the DCIS is spread out or is in more than one location, some women will choose to undergo a mastectomy." I read these 10 pages many times and kept changing my mind about which treatment choice to select. I highly recommend you visit this site. Print it out and read it a few times. You are also likely to change your mind many times before reaching your final treatment decision. The key point is you must select a treatment choice, even for early stage breast cancer.

In addition to my internet research, I began talking to people about my recent diagnosis. My tax preparer connected me with her friend Beth who also had experienced breast cancer and opted to have a double mastectomy. She called me around 9:00 p.m., just before my bedtime. I now regret that I answered her call because after our conversation, she put the fear of God into me and I couldn't fall asleep. Her frightening words echoed in my brain.

Beth initially had a more advanced stage of breast cancer than I had and now had another cancer, deemed terminal. She told me I didn't seem like someone who would want to keep looking in the rearview mirror worrying about whether I would have a recurrence. She talked to me with a directness far different than how the doctors spoke to me. Beth also shared that California state law requires that insurance companies pay for reconstruction after a mastectomy. Although I cringed at the word, I did feel a strange sense of relief.

POINTS FROM DR. BARRY:

- **Federal law requires that your insurance company has to pay for reconstruction after a mastectomy.**

- **Discuss the different methods of reconstruction with your doctor and your insurance company.**

I later spoke to Lila, a business associate's wife and a breast cancer survivor. She had inflammatory breast cancer and had a mastectomy, chemotherapy, and radiation. She had been a radiation technician and gave me some information about radiation. She said that radiation is given with an intention to halt the cancer. Usually women need two to four weeks of healing after lumpectomies before radiation starts. Radiation usually lasts six or seven weeks. The radiation needs to get to a certain dose to get rid of the cancer without damaging the good cells. One must finish the whole course of radiation. She shared that people often do not experience too many side effects. Some common side effects are redness, like a sun burn; and the breast can become hard and shrink.

Paul told a co-worker at his work about my diagnosis which surprised me. He's generally a private man. His co-worker, Cindy, put me in touch with her sister-in-law, Sally, who recently had a double mastectomy. I learned she also had multi focal DCIS and had chosen a double mastectomy instead of radiation and drugs. We began speaking and emailing three weeks after her mastectomies. She seemed to be doing great. Hearing about her story and recovery helped prepare me for what I would face. It did not, however, calm my racing mind.

Sally had worked in the medical field and had done a lot of research to discover the best treatment for multifocal DCIS. Through using different methods, we had both decided that having both breasts removed via a bilateral mastectomy was our best option.

Sally gave me a great suggestion about a special camisole designed for women to wear right after a mastectomy. It is made by a company called Amoena. (www.amoena.com 1(800) 926-6362). It has little pouches attached to the camisole with velcro so you can put your drains in them. (After surgery you will most likely be sent home with a plastic tube or drain in each breast which has been operated on. The drain is gathering fluid and blood that is being released from the site.) Thus, you can go out and not worry about your unattractive drains showing. My surgeon wrote me a prescription for the camisole, and then I picked it up from a medical supply place. Fortunately, my insurance plan paid for it. The doctors and nurses at my insurance plan didn't know about the camisole, so I showed it to them and shared the details. The camisole also comes with two little fiberfill prosthetics in case you want to use them. Each camisole is about $50. I purchased two of them and highly recommend them. You can also find them at Nordstrom's.

During our frequent email exchanges, Sally became a bit too graphic about the downsides of her recovery. I feel bad but, for my own protection I told her not to share these details because I wanted to maintain a positive attitude. I preferred not to focus on what could go wrong with my mastectomies. Our minds can be very interesting. I started doubting my decision. Was this choice too drastic? Sally assured me her recovery was going well, and she thought mastectomies beat the alternatives. I still wasn't 100% sure of what to do.

I spoke to my friend, Maria, whose mother had died of breast cancer. Maria had been diagnosed with atypical cells and had chosen to take Tamoxifen as a preventive measure. She recommended I go to Dr. Susan Love's website, http://www.dslrf.org/breastcancer. I looked at the site, and once again read that for multi focal DCIS the recommended treatment choices are mastectomy or radiation followed by Tamoxifen or other drugs.

While going back and forth about what treatment to get, I started thinking about ladies who had mastectomies. What stood out for me is they were still alive to talk about their breast cancer. I mentioned this to my ex-boyfriend Brian who is a doctor in Georgia. In his supportive way he shared that what I had was very treatable. He suggested I start taking some liquid vitamins and minerals to boost my immune system. He also had me send my pathology reports to him so he could forward them to his brother Rick, the head of oncology in a hospital on the East coast. Rick felt that based on my pathology, I was a good candidate for radiation. Brian encouraged me to remain objective about my breast cancer treatment; however, he also helped remind me I had cancer. This was no research project. My life was at stake and at some point I would have to come to terms that it was really me with the cancer.

Brian agreed that mastectomy is the tried and true treatment for breast cancer. I still can't believe how barbaric this sounds. He commented that if you get cancer in your foot, they may cut it off. One would think in this day and age, with all of the advances we have made as a species, that we would have better solutions than removing body parts. I implore anyone who reads this to find a better solution to cancer for the upcoming generations.

I am not a doctor, and I did not research the current drug choices with great depth. I made the choice that I felt would give me and my family the most secure future.

I discussed my treatment options extensively with my mother, Sandy, who lives with us. In fact, we visited every night in her room to mull over my decisions. From the beginning, she thought the mastectomies were my best choice. Alternatively, I kept going back and forth with my decision. I tried to be objective and pretend that I was doing research for a friend that came to me with a problem. I analyzed the pros and cons of radiation and drugs versus mastectomy.

I had pretty much decided if I opted for a mastectomy I would have a double mastectomy to alleviate future problems. Plus I wanted a matched set of new breasts. My breasts were still attractive yet why match a new breast to a saggy, 41 year old, post- nursing breast. In my head, I had to start thinking that I was just getting a boob job. I thought this might take some of the sting out of my situation. Yet later, when I realized I would lose my nipples, I wasn't sure removing the second breast had been such a good idea.

During my research, I tried to narrow it to a breast cancer diagnosis soon after or during breastfeeding. I clung to the possibility that I had been misdiagnosed because my cells looked different due to breastfeeding. I wondered why women are not supposed to get a mammogram for six months after breastfeeding. It seemed logical to me that our cells could change during and soon after breastfeeding. I still think there could be something to that. Yet I never found anything online or from talking to people to validate a misdiagnosis due to breastfeeding.

I next spoke to one of the head radiologists in my insurance plan, Dr. N. He appreciated my questions yet confirmed breastfeeding would not change my diagnosis. He recommended I speak directly to the pathologists who had examined my breast tissue. Unfortunately, a pathologist's report is subjective. A diagnosis is often not clear cut and, two pathologists can arrive at a different diagnosis. In my case, the first pathologist diagnosed me with DCIS while another pathologist found the second DCIS which made my diagnosis multi focal DCIS. The pathologist I spoke to reviewed my reports, specimens, and confirmed my diagnosis also concluding that breastfeeding did not affect his findings.

Even though I hadn't practiced law in years, I believe my insurance plan's records still listed me as an attorney. During my encounters with the various doctors, I wondered if they were "attorneying" up to me. Since doctors often fear attorneys, maybe this explained the extra time and care they took to answer my questions and make things available to me. This could also explain why no one would tell me which treatment choice would be best for me. Perhaps it could be grounds for me to sue them if I had a recurrence after a treatment option they had recommended. Maybe doctors are so afraid of getting sued for malpractice they don't want to tell the patient what to do. Actually, I think the doctors expect the patient to make the right treatment choice on his/her own. Whatever the case, it is essential to do your own research and make the right decision for yourself.

The general surgeon, Dr. X, called me to re-emphasize that with the second finding of DCIS, I had to make my decision and take action regarding my treatment. She meant a Western Medicine form of treatment.

I learned my insurance plan has a board of doctors whom get together once a week to discuss cases. Dr. X had someone present my case to the board and with my diagnosis and history, they advised either the mastectomy or radiation followed by medication.

POINTS FROM DR. BARRY:

- **This group is called a tumor board.**
- **Most hospitals have a tumor board and it is usually run by an oncologist and includes surgeons, radiologists, pathologists, and other oncologists.**

During our conversation, Dr. X also suggested I get a mammogram. If it returned negative, then I should have an MRI of my breast. If the MRI didn't show anything then she recommended I have the radiation or the mastectomy. If the mammogram or MRI revealed something more serious than DCIS, then I must see another surgeon during her vacation. She further mentioned that even with a mastectomy there would be a very small risk I could get breast cancer again because a bit of tissue is left behind. Also, if I chose reconstruction I may be able to do it simultaneous with the mastectomies or at a later date. (Simultaneous means that the reconstruction process would begin during the mastectomies yet would be a several month step-by-step process.) We also discussed taking off my other breast as a preventive measure. Dr. X thought if they only found DCIS then "the most definitive treatment" would be mastectomy and no lymph nodes would need to be taken out. Further, I would most likely not need hormone therapy, radiation, or chemotherapy if they only found DCIS, and I had a double mastectomy. Thus, I would be done with treatment. (I didn't know that she also felt I would be done with follow-up as I will explain later.)

Dr. X suggested I see a radiation therapist, oncologist and plastic surgeon to help with my decision making. This sounded more serious. I asked about the gene test I had heard about, and Dr. X offered to refer me to genetics for the test. She mentioned if the test came back positive for the gene mutation then I would have an 86% chance of getting breast cancer. Given this high probability, she would then recommend I have a bilateral mastectomy and also have my ovaries removed as well. No one had recommended I take this test. In retrospect, I would rather have met with the genetic counselor and taken the gene test during my initial testing. It would have helped me to make my decision for treatment straight away.

Cutting off a breast may not seem like "treatment" yet, unfortunately, it is still one of our best choices, even for early stage breast cancer. You may want to consider getting the BRCA1 and BRCA2 gene mutation blood test if you have close relatives who have had breast cancer, are of Ashkenazi Jewish descent, or if you are grappling over a treatment option after a breast cancer diagnosis. So you are aware, I will discuss this test in much further detail later in this book.

During my research I realized if I had radiation and then had a recurrence in that breast, I would most likely be forced to get a mastectomy because one can't get radiation in the same area of the breast twice. Dr. X. confirmed this. Plus, if you have had radiation and then need a mastectomy; you may not be able to have reconstruction. If you can have reconstruction, you may need back flap or TRAM flap reconstruction, or you may be able to choose expanders with implants. However, the results of any method of reconstruction may not turn out as well due to the previous radiation. As you can see, this information is really important to know about before you make a treatment decision.

POINTS FROM DR. BARRY:

- **You can have complications with any method of reconstruction.**
- **Expanders with implants are not necessarily less complicated than the TRAM flap or back flap methods of reconstruction.**

I spoke to my friend, Connie, who had breast cancer and radiation treatment a few years before my diagnosis. She had radiation five days a week for seven weeks. She didn't consider the radiation unpleasant, but it really hit her a few weeks into the treatment and zapped her energy. She shared that if she had it to do over she would have opted for the mastectomy. The radiation had shrunk her breast and made it very misshaped. She did not tolerate Tamoxifen well, so she took a different medication, Arimidex. Even though Connie is a well-educated woman, I am not certain she researched her choices well-enough. She may have selected what she thought would be the easiest treatment.

Then I spoke to Paul's Aunt Jean. She had breast cancer and radiation many years ago and also said her breast shrunk. One of these ladies referred to her boob as a "raisin breast." My internet research didn't seem to make radiation a negative option but from what I heard from the ladies, it didn't seem very appealing.

May 30, 2006

I met with an Oncologist, Dr. P, which my friend, Connie, had recommended. I prepared a list of questions for him. I found many of them on the internet site: www.getbcfacts.com. I used the area called, "Questions for your doctor," and took out the questions I thought were most important. The main categories are questions about diagnosis, tumor testing, surgery, radiation therapy, chemotherapy and hormonal treatment. View the site and select the questions that you want answers to. To make an informed decision which is right for you, I recommend that you learn as much about breast cancer and your treatment choices as you can. Don't overwhelm yourself but educate yourself.

Before meeting with the oncologist, Paul thought I was nuts when I told him based on my research, my recommended treatment would likely be a mastectomy. He told me I'd over-reacted and suggested I wait to hear what the oncologist had to say. My mom, Paul and I met with Dr. P at his office. He told us my cancer was in the duct and not in the fat. Thus, it generally doesn't spread. Removing the cancer would be curative. With DCIS I have a higher risk of developing more serious, invasive breast cancer. Based on my diagnosis of multi focal DCIS (two separate areas of ductal carcinoma in situ that were not connected), my age (41), and ethnicity (Ashkenazi-meaning that my ancestors were Jewish and from Eastern Europe), the recommended treatments were mastectomy or radiation followed by Tamoxifen. The radiation would be administered to my whole breast. Then he shared his best news. I wouldn't die from this cancer diagnosis.

Dr. P initially told me if I only choose radiation, I would then have a 13.4% chance of a recurrence of breast cancer within 5 years and there would be a 6.7% probability that it would be invasive cancer, as well as a 6.7% possibility it would be non-invasive cancer. Essentially I'd have a 50% chance of having invasive cancer if I had a recurrence of breast cancer. (He called me on June 1, 2006 to change his numbers after he spoke to the Radiologist, Dr. T about my situation. Instead of 13.4% it became a 9% chance of a recurrence within 5 years with a 4.5% probability of being invasive and a 4.5% chance it would be non-invasive cancer.) If I had radiation followed by Tamoxifen it would cut my risk to an 8.2% chance of re-emergence within 5 years with a 4.1% chance it would return as invasive cancer and 4.1% possibility it would come back as non-invasive cancer. (He also modified these numbers in the later telephone call to a 6% chance of a recurrence within 5 years with a 3% risk that it would be invasive cancer.) Getting a double mastectomy would give me a 0-1% chance of getting breast cancer again. I liked these odds better than the risk of recurrence if I chose radiation followed by drugs.

Not getting treatment at all gave me a 33% chance I would have breast cancer in either breast. I wouldn't accept this option. These statistics didn't take into account that I may have the BRCA gene mutation. If positive for the gene then I would have over a 50% chance of getting cancer again. I don't know exactly how Dr. P and Dr. T arrived at their numbers, yet it is important to have some trust with what our doctors tell us. Being a numbers person, I primarily based my decision on the chance of recurrence with each treatment choice. Given the above numbers, I had no more interest in meeting with Dr. T, the Radiologist. My statistics were all I needed.

If the numbers are not enough for you, then you may want to meet with the radiation people for their input. Keep in mind that a Radiologist will probably think their treatment is the best choice, as will a Surgeon, and so on. This is their work specialty where they focus their attention and belief. Make the decision which is right for you!

Dr. P indicated it is impossible to know if a recurrence will come back as non-invasive or invasive cancer until it occurs. For some women the DCIS will never become invasive yet for others it will. There is no way to predict what can happen if DCIS is left un-treated. It can metastasize over a number of years. They just don't know which women will have DCIS that never becomes more than DCIS and which women will have DCIS that becomes invasive and when it will do that. Although I did not know what the outcome would be if I didn't treat my cancer, I did find out later my cancer had been deemed "high grade" which meant if it did return, it would do so aggressively.

As mentioned, during my internet research I found some great sites (see appendix) which listed questions to ask the different doctors. One question that I asked my oncologist, Dr. P, "If I were your daughter, would you suggest a mastectomy or radiation? He replied, "That is a hard question." He never gave me a straight answer. He suggested I consider the risk I'd be willing to live with and to think about how I'd feel if there was an "abnormality."

Again, I found it interesting that none of my doctors would clearly tell me what to do. I had to pursue my answers and make my choices. As I've mentioned before, doctors don't really seem to want to go out on a limb to help us make decisions. They merely provide information, and we are expected to know what our best choices are. You may encounter this same situation, and have to pursue answers and make an informed decision as to which treatment choice is best for you. I hope this book helps you to make the best decision for yourself.

Dr. P recommended I get a mammogram and then an MRI. If they didn't find any more cancer then radiation and Tamoxifen might be effective. He also shared at my age, 41, Tamoxifen shouldn't increase the risk of uterine cancer. However, Tamoxifen could launch me into menopause, increase my chance of osteoporosis, and slightly enhance the possibility of blood clots. Taking Vitamin D and calcium would help decrease the potential risks. He said radiation would be six to seven weeks. When I asked about the side effects from radiation, he told me I could expect fatigue, inflammation of the skin, and some shrinking of the breast. I asked him if Tamoxifen would prevent cancer in other body parts, and he said "no." If this drug could prevent cancer in other areas of my body, the radiation/Tamoxifen choice would have been more attractive to me.

Dr. P indicated a mastectomy with immediate reconstruction would take about a month to recover from. He said I could most likely get immediate reconstruction and recommended I speak to the plastic surgeon about implants versus the TRAM flap procedure. I asked him if I should have my lymph nodes tested and he commented that this is usually not done with DCIS. If they found invasive cancer then a radioactive tracer would be placed in my breast.

Honestly, I didn't know what all of this meant but was glad that I had some questions that I had pulled from the internet. After going through this whole breast cancer thing, reading about breast cancer, researching it, talking to Doctors and other people about breast cancer, I can only tell you that my understanding and knowledge of breast cancer is just the tip of the iceberg. But, I do know more than most people do about breast cancer and more than I thought I would ever know about it. I wrote this book to share the information I gathered with you and save you some research time.

The amount of material about breast cancer seems to be endless. When doing your research be sure and think about the source that you are getting your information from. Do not trust everything you read or see. Be very cautious of strange products that are supposedly going to cure your cancer. Personally, I believe that the Western medicine treatments for breast cancer are still our best choices but have no problem adding in alternative treatment choices to supplement the traditional Western medicine choices.

I asked Dr. P if having multiple biopsies increased my risk of having breast cancer. He said I had an increased risk of breast cancer because the breast was abnormal, not due to the biopsies. I also asked if breastfeeding Andrew right up until the biopsies would change the diagnosis. He did not believe so. I had Andrew's cord blood frozen upon his birth and still pay a yearly fee to maintain this. (I use Cord Blood Registry at 1888 CORDBLOOD. Please mention my name so I can get a free month if you decide to use their service.) I asked if Andrew's stem cells could help me, and Dr. P said "no." I told him since being diagnosed with breast cancer, I felt tired and nauseous. I wondered if these symptoms were just in my head. I figured having breast cancer gave me permission to not feel well. He confirmed that the symptoms were in my head, there should be no symptoms with a diagnosis of DCIS.

I told Dr. P that I had scheduled a mammogram the next day and then would possibly have an MRI. (Keep in mind that I had just stopped breastfeeding less than a month before and had been told earlier that I could not get a mammogram until six months after breastfeeding.) He said that a MRI is more sensitive and that a mammogram misses 15-20% of breast cancer. Isn't that comforting?

Then I told him I might be getting a referral to be tested for the BRCA gene. He said I must attend an educational program before having the test. He didn't discuss whether or not I should have the test. Again, in retrospect, I believe that had he or Dr. X highly suggested I have the gene test, this would have made my decision much easier, as well as, wiser. If I am positive for the gene mutation then I certainly would have had a double mastectomy. (See the gene mutation discussion starting on page 138.)

I asked Dr. P how to build my immune system. He suggested a good diet with more grains, fruit, vegetables, fish, and less red meat. He also recommended I take Vitamin D and calcium supplements, get exercise, and rest.

He told me he'd be away on vacation but that he'd return at the end of June. He suggested I visit the website: www.cancer.gov to see the following study: NSABP B24.

During our phone conversation when he called me to adjust the statistics he had given me, Dr. P indicated the "standard approach" for my diagnosis is mastectomy. Again, he didn't say that he would recommend a mastectomy. What does "standard approach" mean?

POINTS FROM DR. BARRY:

- **Standard approach implies the standard of care. Anything less can be construed as malpractice.**

Dr. P also stated I had the cancer for awhile, "probably" years. It probably wouldn't have shown up on a mammogram and the little lump I had felt in my breast was "probably" not related to the DCIS. He also shared it would "probably" be okay to take my August trip to Italy that I had booked and paid for many months ago and delay put off my treatment until my return. In looking at my notes, I notice many "probably's." I wanted to eliminate as many "probably's" as possible.

I opted for a bilateral or as I prefer to call it, double mastectomy. I wanted to minimize my future risks and not live in fear of a recurrence. Bottom line, with two small children I want to be alive to take care of them and also, for my own sake. A double mastectomy gave me the best chance of survival, at least from my point of view, along with the least chance of recurrence.

When making a treatment decision please consider which treatment choice will give you the best chance of survival and the least chance of recurrence while also taking into consideration the side effects you may encounter from each treatment. Consider this my golden nugget to you in what I believe is the best way to make your treatment choice.

The four months I experienced from my diagnosis in May of 2006 until my mastectomies in September 2006, were the most stressful period of my life thus far. I could barely sleep at night. I would try Xanax, Tylenol P.M. or Excedrin P.M. to get to sleep. During the day I sometimes took Xanax to help lessen my anxiety.

I did more research on the internet about my treatment options. According to the National Cancer Institute website http://www.cancer. gov/cancertopics/breast-cancer-surgery-choices, most women who have DCIS or Stage I, IIA, IIB, or IIIA breast cancer have three basic SURGERY choices. They are 1) breast-sparing surgery 2) mastectomy, or 3) mastectomy with breast reconstruction surgery. Please see Section "D" of this book for more information on mastectomies and reconstruction. Section "D" starts on page 177.

It perplexed me that these were my only choices for treating early stage breast cancer. I thought with more research I would find a better treatment choice. I did my research with relentless fury but, sadly, could not find a better treatment choice.

June 2, 2006

Mom, baby Andrew, and I met with Dr. S, the reconstruction surgeon. Of all of the doctors I have seen, he was the most helpful in influencing my treatment decision. He is very kind, caring, and compassionate. Thankfully, he turned out to be quite skilled. We reviewed my diagnosis, I cried, and he gave me Kleenex.

Right before we met with the doctor, we watched a movie about mastectomies; the different methods of reconstruction and information from women who had mastectomies. Actually, Andrew acted up and I don't remember much about that movie. I did take notes, so I will share those with you as well as other information I have gathered on reconstruction in Section "D" of this book. I will also share what I personally experienced during my reconstruction. (Taking notes is just part of my training, even when my brain doesn't remember what I wrote down.)

During my meeting with Dr. S, I told him that if I chose to have a mastectomy, I would want a double mastectomy. I didn't see a point in matching my 41-year-old saggy boob which had just finished breastfeeding; and I feared getting breast cancer in my other breast. I asked him if he could give me two new 20-year-old boobs. He replied, "We will work on them until we are both happy." While crying I said, "You are the man for me." I felt very good about my meeting with Dr.

S. He really was the first doctor who told me he thought a bilateral mastectomy "wasn't a bad decision," and that he had performed reconstruction on other women with similar diagnoses to mine, who had decided to have both breasts removed.

Dr. S said that Dr. X would perform a skin sparing mastectomy and remove my areola and my nipples (again I had this in my notes but didn't realize until much later that I would be losing my nipples) but would leave a lot of my own skin. Dr. S would then put the breast tissue expanders in to stretch my skin, close me up, and leave a drain on each side. At the time of surgery, he would put in as much saline as possible into the expanders/temporary implants, and then he would gradually fill the expanders over the next two months. After that I would return to the operating room where he would release some of the scar tissue and put in my permanent implants. About two months later I would go to the surgery room at his office where he would create nipples with my skin. About two weeks after that he would tattoo me. I had faith in Dr. S and knew he would do the best he could to give me two great breasts. He did mention a downside with the implants as being my new breasts would be very firm, and I could have wrinkling. He was right because my reconstructed boobs are a little softer than softballs, and I do have some ridges. But they look great in clothes.

I learned from Dr. S that most of the recovery from the first surgery would be from the mastectomies and not from the expanders and I should not do heavy lifting for several weeks after the surgery. He also said that after the mastectomies, I might have drains in for about two weeks. He would put catheters in that dripped anesthesia directly to the site for pain control for a few days. He then said I'd either go home the day of my surgery or stay overnight in the hospital. I informed him I would stay in the hospital for a night or two, and I would not have this surgery on an outpatient basis. (I highly recommend that you consider staying in the hospital for a night or two after a mastectomy. I don't recommend going through this on an outpatient basis. You will not feel great and may need nursing care.) He agreed and arranged to be my discharge doctor since he would close me up. He said the other procedures could be done on an outpatient basis but someone must drive me home.

We also discussed the other methods of reconstruction briefly. I learned the TRAMflap method (which uses tissue from your stomach) would not be a good choice for me because it wouldn't give me much tissue to create breasts; and it could decrease my abdominal muscle strength. He said it is a major surgery, so there is a chance the newly created breast flap will not survive. Dr. S said the back flap method was used primarily for women who previously had radiation to their breast.

When deciding which procedure is right for you, try to get the best information possible and don't overanalyze everything (like me). Make the best decision for you - not for your doctor or significant other. Really think about the risks you are willing to live with, what procedure gives you the best chance of survival and the least chance of recurrence. Do not just pick the procedure that sounds easiest.

I had an appointment scheduled to meet with radiation professionals. After meeting with Dr. S, researching, talking to people, and evaluating the situation, I decided to cancel it. I didn't want to get swayed from my decision to have a bilateral mastectomy.

After meeting with the doctors and doing my research, I realized if I had the mastectomies and they found no invasive cancer, I would not need any further treatment. Thus, no medication, radiation or chemotherapy would be necessary.

On the other hand, if I chose radiation there would be a greater chance during the course of my life to get breast cancer again in either breast. If I had a recurrence, I would need to have treatment again. If breast cancer developed in my right breast again after having radiation, I would most likely need a mastectomy anyway. It would be unlikely that they could radiate the same breast again, since I was told that I would need to have to have my whole right breast radiated, thus the need for a mastectomy would be my only option for a recurrence in that breast.

Even years later following my bilateral mastectomies, I still worry about the possibility of a recurrence. I don't know what is going on in my breasts since I can't get a mammogram or ultrasound because there is little or no tissue to view. Even though I have lowered my risk of getting breast cancer significantly, if I do have a recurrence, I want to find it quickly. Yet I've been so displeased with the lack of follow-up for a possible recurrence. My only follow-up has been a physical breast examination by a doctor or other medical provider. I do emphasize that even with the limits in follow-up available to me, I am still happy with my decision to have a bilateral mastectomy. Although my fear of a recurrence has not completely gone away, it no longer keeps me awake at night and it is not what I focus on. My life is much calmer than during those four months between my diagnosis and my mastectomies. I now rarely worry about breast cancer returning because I know I have done so much to reduce my risk of a recurrence.

Soon after meeting with Dr. S on June 2, 2006, I scheduled my bilateral mastectomies and reconstructive surgeries for July 10th. Once I made the decision to have the surgery, I wanted to schedule it right away, yet I had to coordinate a date between two surgeons and that wasn't easy. Also, we had paid for a trip to Italy leaving on August 11th. I longed to have the surgeries behind me. I told Gabby, my then ten-year-old daughter, I would have the surgery and try my best to go on our trip a month later. If I wasn't feeling well enough, we must postpone our trip. She burst out crying. I didn't know what to do. We talked about it and she was mainly afraid for her mom- not being a spoiled brat crying over a trip. It will never be a good time to have your breasts removed. Somehow, if you need major surgery, you just have to muster up the strength, schedule it, and show up.

POINTS FROM DR. BARRY:

- **Illness often gets in the way of our lives.**
- **It can be difficult to coordinate two surgeons.**

June of 2006

I am a very open person and discuss what is going on in my life with many people. I mentioned my breast cancer to Sheila, a colleague who helped me do my escrows for my mortgage business. Interestingly enough, she brought me some information on the HALO NAF breast cancer screening test. It mentioned that the HALO NAF Breast PAP test can detect early abnormal breast cancer CELLS possibly seven or eight years before a mammogram can detect a lump. (Mammograms don't look at cells.) Thus, the HALO NAF test may be able to find abnormal cells during their pre-invasive stage. The five minute test is done in the doctor's office. Suction cups, like breast pumps used during breastfeeding, are attached to each breast. The breast is compressed and light suction is applied to bring nipple fluid to the surface. The fluid is collected and sent to the laboratory for analysis. Please see more discussion of the HALO NAF test in the sections of this book called "Pregnancy" and "Screening Tests." See pages 113 and 159.

I read in the literature that Dr. Baxter-Jones, M.D., M.B.A, a board-certified Obstetrician/Gynecologist was not too far from my house. She had been distinguished as the first physician in the country to use this FDA approved test. I called Dr. Baxter-Jones' office (858-592-6299) to find out more about the test. I learned the test costs $95 and if fluid is produced, it gets analyzed for an additional $45. I would have taken the test but I was told that I could not get the test until three to six months after I finished breastfeeding, preferably six months. I didn't want to delay my mastectomies just for this test although I wondered if it would find abnormal cells in my breasts. Looking back I wish I had talked to Dr. Baxter-Jones about getting the test, even though I had recently been breastfeeding. Since my breasts would soon be taken off, the HALO NAF results could have been easily compared to what was actually found in my breasts when they were analyzed after my mastectomies. This may have provided a learning experience for researchers.

Please go to the websites: www.paptestforthebreast.com and www.neomatrix.com for more information on this test. You can also call 1800 628-2880 to find out more. This FDA approved test may not be available in your area yet and may not be covered by your insurance.

If you have breast cancer you want to catch it as early as possible. Some believe breast cancer moves across a spectrum. It is thought that 95%, if not all, of breast cancer starts in the ducts. The cancer starts within a normal duct, then can become hyperplasia, then Atypical Ductal Hyperplasia, you then may move on to Ductal Carcinoma in Situ and, if not detected, you may move on to Invasive Ductal Carcinoma.

POINTS FROM DR. BARRY:

- **Invasive Ductal Carcinoma is the same as Infiltrating Ductal Carcinoma.**

A biopsy revealed I was in the Atypical Ductal Hyperplasia stage at the end of 1998. The mammogram did not detect it. Maybe I could have done something to prevent moving along the spectrum, but my doctors did not suggest anything, nor did I know what to do at that time.

By 2006 I had multi focal (found in more than one spot) Ductal Carcinoma in Situ. Again, this was not seen in my mammogram. A biopsy discovered it. I was not going to wait around to have the cancer move along the spectrum and make it all the way to Invasive Ductal Carcinoma. No one wants cancer at all, yet I feel fortunate to have found my cancer at an early stage.

A little chart in the literature given to me about the HALO NAF test (See my sections on Pregnancy and Screening tests for more information.) sent me into a tailspin. It states that "Diagnosis of breast cancer within two years of child birth has close to a 50% mortality rate." This came from "The Relation of Reproductive Factors to Mortality from Breast Cancer" and is found in Cancer Epidemiology Biomarkers and Prevention, Volume 11, pages 235-241 from March of 2002. Janet R. Daling Kathleen E. Malone, David R. Doody, Benjamin O. Anderson and Peggy L. Porter wrote the article.

I located this article on the internet (see http://cebp.aacrjournals.org/cgi/content/abstract/11/3/235) and read the study.

Learning that 48.2% of women die after being diagnosed with breast cancer within two years of having a child, disturbed me. I spoke to my doctor friend, Brian, about it. He reminded me they said "INVASIVE" breast cancer. My cancer was not invasive. I felt a little better yet still upset. Be careful with the information you come across.

I'm sure the lady who gave me the HALO -NAF packet meant to be helpful. She must not have noticed the little box which mentioned having a new baby and the increased mortality from breast cancer. It stood out for me since I had recently been diagnosed with breast cancer and had just stopped nursing my 17 month old son. Thus, I had a baby within two years of being diagnosed with breast cancer. Thankfully, my cancer did not turn out to be invasive. I beg you to take this warning and statistic seriously. If your doctor thinks your breast problem is just an infection or something minor, make sure he/she is absolutely right, especially if you had a baby within the last two years. This could cost you your life if they are wrong.

I looked at another article, "Effect of reproductive factors on stage, grade and hormone receptor status in early-onset breast cancer," by Joan A. Largent, Argyrios Ziogas and Hoda Anton-Culver, written in 2005. It can be found online at: http://breast-cancer-research.com/content/7/4/R541. (See this study and my section on Pregnancy. This is very important information.)

In writing this book, I came up with more questions than answers. Does not getting your period mean you aren't producing certain hormones, i.e. estrogen? Is the less estrogen you produce better in terms of not getting breast cancer? Maybe that is why women who start their periods at a young age may have a higher risk for breast cancer. It could be that it isn't so much the age you began your period but the length of time your body has produced certain hormones. I am definitely not a doctor or a scientist. This may be common knowledge but, if so, I am unaware of it. I started writing this book with a lot of questions, and as I have progressed I've noticed I have even more questions. Thankfully, my diligent research led to some answers and a basic understanding of breast cancer. You will need to keep reading to get my laypersons interpretation of the interplay of estrogen, pregnancy, and other factors on your likelihood of getting breast cancer.

I next looked at my brochure about gene testing which I will go into more detail about later, and I noticed taking oral contraceptives decreases one's risk of ovarian cancer substantially. It does not mention that it decreases the risk of breast cancer. One would think that the "pill" changes hormones thus would produce less estrogen. So, wouldn't this decrease the risk of breast cancer?

I believe controlling estrogen is one of the major keys to preventing and/or controlling breast cancer.

POINTS FROM DR. BARRY:

- **Obesity increases the amount of estrogen in the body.**
- **Obesity and increased estrogen may increase the risk of breast cancer.**

Please read my discussion of Estrogen later in this book.

According to the National Cancer Institute website: http://www.cancer.gov/cancertopics/aromatase-inhibitors, "Many breast tumors are 'estrogen sensitive', meaning the hormone, estrogen, helps them to grow. Aromatase Inhibitors can help block the growth of these tumors by lowering the amount of estrogen in the body. Estrogen is produced by the ovaries and other tissues of the body, using a substance called aromatase." So, if estrogen is produced by the ovaries it makes sense that removing your ovaries decreases your risk of breast cancer if you are premenopausal. (See my discussion of this under the Gene testing section of this book.) Did you know that your ovaries are a main source of your estrogen production before menopause? I didn't realize it until writing this book. Maybe facts like this are common knowledge but I have to admit that I don't know all that I should about the human body.

To return to my story, Dr. X had been on vacation most of June. After my diagnosis of DCIS she told me the board had agreed for me to have a mammogram. I also planned to have a genetic test, as I mentioned earlier, to see if I am genetically pre-disposed to having breast cancer. The test looks at the BRCA1 and BRCA2 genes. I later learned having this gene mutation means one is at a higher risk for breast and ovarian cancer. (I'll share more about this later.) If I had the gene mutation, then I would definitely have the mastectomies. I delayed the test for some time because I feared my young daughter may also be at risk of breast cancer. I hope there will be better treatment choices, if not a cure, when she becomes a woman. Don't we all.

I also wasn't prepared to have my ovaries taken out if my results came back positive for the mutation. By getting my results I might find out information I didn't want to know. Opting for genetic testing is something you must figure out for yourself. If you decide to do the testing, you must be prepared to take action on the results you receive.

More questions came to mind. Why aren't we hearing more about the BRCA1 and BRCA2 gene mutation and the easy blood test (now in 2010 I have learned you can take the test by submitting your saliva) which can detect it? Must we seek out information? What is our role versus the doctor's role? What if we don't ask the right questions or make the right choices? Are doctors too afraid of malpractice suits to actually speak up and tell their patients what the best treatment is for their diagnosis?

This whole breast cancer thing took over my life. Scheduling tests, meeting with different doctors, having tests, biopsies, talking to people, doing research, trying to figure out what to do; a good portion of my every day focused on breast cancer. If you have been diagnosed with breast cancer, you know exactly what I mean.

Although, my insurance plan has a "breast coordinator", they weren't very helpful. They attempted to answer my questions when I phoned, yet overall I felt left on my own. Had I done nothing with my diagnosis, I doubt anyone from my HMO would have pursued me, so I'd begin my treatment. I took the responsibility to be my own advocate. My insurance plan didn't seem to have any set protocols on how to deal with a diagnosis of breast cancer.

This concerns me about women who are not as aggressive as I am or who are afraid to ask questions. What happens to them? Are they the ones still dying of breast cancer? Is there a national or international protocol and standard of care for handling breast cancer? I finally discovered one exists after my treatment choices though I'm grateful I can share this with you.

For a pretty straight forward guideline or standard of care regarding cancer in general and specifically different types of breast cancer, please see the National Comprehensive Cancer Network, NCCN, website at: www.nccn.org. Click on "NCCN Clinical Practice Guidelines in Oncology" and then go to your particular type of breast cancer. You can also go into "patients" and then "guidelines." The first site seems more for medical professionals but both seemed fairly easy to navigate and understand.

Back to my insurance plan stating I couldn't get a mammogram while breastfeeding, or within six months of breastfeeding. Somehow now that I had been diagnosed with breast cancer, they allowed the mammogram even though I had just stopped breastfeeding. This still doesn't make sense to me.

They scheduled me for an evening mammogram. My mother came with me to my appointment, and they told us they could do my mammogram; however, due to my diagnosis, I must come back during the day to meet with a radiologist who could read my mammogram right away. The technician felt upset that the person who scheduled me hadn't realized my diagnosis and situation. I decided to have the mammogram since I was already there. Given my recent surgeries, it hurt to get the mammogram, yet the technician was gentle with me. If you need a mammogram, don't be scared, it does not take very long and it shouldn't be too uncomfortable.

The technician looked at my results of my mammogram and said I must come back to speak with the radiologist. I noticed how upset she seemed. I assured her it was okay. I knew my diagnosis; and most likely I'd have a double mastectomy. Two female technicians were in the room. They hugged me, told me how strong I am, and let me know this was the right decision. Tears were sliding down their faces as they spoke to me. Then they shared about a coworker who felt so challenged after her radiation and other treatment. I found it interesting that technicians and nurses were more willing to voice their opinions than most of the doctors.

POINTS FROM DR. BARRY:

- **Technicians and nurses don't have the ultimate responsibility for patients.**

During my mammogram my mother spoke with another woman in the waiting area. Gabby and I joke that there is no such thing as a "stranger" to my mother. She will talk to anyone and usually hear their life story within five minutes. When I finished with my mammogram, my mom and this woman were still talking. The lady began speaking to me with tears brimming in her eyes. I knew then my mom had told her about my diagnosis. This human compassion touched me. A stranger could be so caring. The lady went in for her mammogram and so did my mom. I overheard the technician say to the lady "You love your breasts, don't you?" and the lady began giggling.

You know I loved my breasts too. In their day they were perky, the right size for my body, and still looked great for being 41-years-old, especially for having nursed two kids. But the quality of my life means more than my breasts. I love my life, as I'd imagine you do yours. If you are diagnosed with breast cancer or some other illness, be smart and do your homework thoroughly. Select the option with the best long-term results for your life. Do not choose "the easy way out." Gather information, talk to people and make an informed decision that is best for you. Don't be afraid to lose your breasts if this is the right choice for you. It is better to lose your breasts than your life.

POINTS FROM DR. BARRY:

- **If you get a diagnosis of breast cancer or some other illness, be smart, really do your homework and pick the option that will give you the best long-term results.**

As the technician predicted, I did need to schedule more mammograms and meet with a radiologist. The Radiologist, Dr. S, showed me my mammogram from three years previously alongside the ones from 2006. In 2003 my mammograms appeared clean but in 2006 both breasts were loaded with calcifications. The calcifications looked like little white spots. Dr. S did not think my breastfeeding skewed the results of my mammograms in any way.

June 21, 2006

I phoned Dr. L, one of the pathologists who gave me the diagnosis. I still thought my breast tissue looked different because of my recent breastfeeding, so I wanted to ensure they knew I had breastfed right up until the time of my biopsies. He mentioned lactation changes the surrounding breast, and breast tissue is stimulated by breastfeeding and pregnancy. Cells do look different when one breastfeeds and the epithelial cells can develop exaggerated abnormal features. However, abnormal cells are abnormal and will continue to progress along the path of being abnormal. They do not improve or return to being normal cells. He said that I had high-grade DCIS, ductal carcinoma in situ; and my recent breastfeeding had no bearing on the diagnosis. He shared that he understood my concern, then agreed to review the slides again and promised to call back with his findings. He also said I could take the slides for another opinion. Dr. L called me back after he re-analyzed my cells and showed them to a group of pathologists. He confirmed my diagnosis of high grade multifocal DCIS.

To digress somewhat from my chronology of events, I began noticing how the right people seemed to show up in my life to support me. On September 29, 2007, a year after my mastectomies, I boarded a 6:20 a.m. flight from San Diego to Chicago to attend my 25th high school reunion. Since my 15 year law school reunion in San Diego had been held the night before, and I didn't care to miss either one, this early flight became my only option. I sat on the aisle while an older gentleman (in his 80's) had the window seat. We had no one in between us, and I planned to sleep right through the flight. Before I could doze off, the older man struck up a conversation with me and after awhile I no longer cared about my rest. Ironically, Dr. M had worked as a pathologist. Although retired, he was headed to Chicago for a pathology convention. He told me hearing about recent advancements in pathology kept his mind sharp.

I soon felt like a reporter sitting with my new interviewee, Dr. M. I told him about my being a breast cancer survivor, and about writing a book on my experience with breast cancer. I shared the abbreviated version of my story. I requested his permission to ask him some work-related questions. He agreed. I first asked, "Would my recent breastfeeding before my cancer diagnosis have any bearing on the diagnosis?"

He paused for a few seconds and then replied, "No, breastfeeding would not change the diagnosis."

I then asked, "Does having multiple biopsies promote cancer?"

He replied, "No, multiple biopsies would not cause cells to turn to cancer."

Dr. M also said DCIS is difficult to find, and he confirmed I had made the right choice, especially by removing the other breast which had an increased risk for breast cancer.

Somehow, we talked for four hours on all kinds of topics and later became email buddies. He referred me to an informative website: www.mybiopsy.org and sent me an e-mail with this excerpt: "DCIS can be cured by a local wide excision. (For some of us smaller breasted women, a wide excision can be fairly close to having a mastectomy.)

A woman who wants to keep her breast and is willing to gamble that a recurrence can be found on a timely basis before it has spread, without obsessing or worrying, should follow this course. On the other hand, if one is going to be worried or obsessed about the possibility of a recurrence, then psychologically and medically one is better off with mastectomies to be free from worry about cancer of the breast." I would have been one of the women who worried non-stop about a recurrence if I had not had both of my breasts removed.

June 26, 2006

Now we return to my situation at pre-surgery when the Surgeon, Dr. X, called me. She had returned from her vacation and noticed I had been scheduled for a bilateral mastectomy on July 10, 2006. Before the surgery she wanted me to have a stereotactic, needle biopsy, to take out the most suspicious calcifications which had appeared on my mammogram. The number of calcifications on my mammogram must have surprised her.

I didn't understand why I needed more biopsies/surgeries if my boobs were coming off anyway. Yet Dr. X explained she wanted to know if there was anything worse than DCIS before she did my surgery. She needed as much information beforehand as possible so she didn't encounter anything unusual, and, also, so she could plan everything out before the surgery. If I only had DCIS, and nothing worse she would do a sentinel node dissection and, thus, take only a few lymph nodes. If I had something worse then she would need to take out more lymph nodes. She wasn't certain; however, if the sentinel node biopsy would work on my right side because of all my previous biopsies. If they only found DCIS or benign tissue in the stereotactic biopsies and if she couldn't find the sentinel node, she would just stop at that point. If they found invasive cancer during the new biopsy then she would have to do more; she didn't specify what "more" would be. Did I understand all of this at the time? Certainly not. My head was spinning with all of this information.

Then Dr. X affirmed my decision to have a bilateral mastectomy stating it as "a very reasonable choice based on my mammogram." She told me that even with mastectomies, a few breast cells would be left behind, and that we would need to continue to feel the breast area for abnormalities. We discussed whether I should have the surgery in July or wait until September, so I could go to Italy in August. We decided if the new biopsies were negative, or if they showed more DCIS, we would wait until September for the mastectomies. If they found invasive cancer, then I would schedule the surgery on July 10th as planned. I really hadn't thought about having a more serious cancer until now. I felt my heart beating faster. Now I had even more to worry about, and I caught my mind wandering to all the "what if's." Then I re-focused my mind on my diagnosis being early stage, non-invasive breast cancer, the original finding. Thankfully, this turned out to be the case.

Going back over our earlier conversation, I had to look up "sentinel node biopsy." According to the National Cancer Institutes' website a sentinel lymph node biopsy is the "Removal and examination of the sentinel node(s), the first lymph node(s) to which cancer cells are likely to spread from a primary tumor. To identify the sentinel lymph node(s), the surgeon injects a radioactive substance, blue dye, or both near the tumor. The surgeon then uses a scanner to find the sentinel lymph node(s) containing the radioactive substance or looks for the lymph node(s) stained with dye. The surgeon then removes the sentinel node(s) to check for the presence of cancer cells."

Ask your doctors to explain terms or procedures that you do not understand and/or look them up by using a reputable source of information.

June 27, 2006

I called radiology and they got me in for my stereotactic biopsies the following day. I wondered why they were able to schedule me so soon since I knew this wasn't typical. Were things worse than what the doctors had told me? I asked myself. There are so many unknowns when one goes through something like this. Even with the improved testing and screening that we now have, doctors don't always know what you have until they open you up, biopsy your tissue, and analyze your situation.

June 28, 2006

My niece, Samantha, drove me to the hospital for the stereotactic biopsies. I would have driven myself but she insisted on taking me to my appointment. I didn't think this biopsy would be a big deal. It was. The technician, Vicky, who performed most of the procedure, was kind. We spoke for about an hour or more based on her taking a look at my recent mammogram. She shared what this test might reveal, how I now had an extreme amount of calcifications in both breasts, and that she often handled difficult cases. She assured me that she'd been doing this work for a long time and could often find things that other people could not. We discussed treatment choices. I told I was leaning toward getting a double mastectomy. Based on her experience and what she saw in my chart and mammogram, she thought it was a good idea.

Vicky also helped influence me to choose mastectomies rather than radiation and drugs. She told me since I had so many calcifications she would only take samples of the ones which seemed the most suspicious I recall the radiologist being in the room some of that time, and also, how I felt Vicky, the technician, seemed more experienced and personable than this doctor.

POINTS FROM DR. BARRY:

- **A radiologist is a doctor.**

I agreed to have as many samples taken as possible. I had already been scheduled for the mastectomies, yet I still wanted as much evidence as possible to confirm my decision. I am an attorney so of course I like evidence.

They first had me lie on a table face down with my breast through a hole in the table. Vicky observed my breast on a computer screen while the doctor and/or Vicky directed a needle to a suspicious area. They froze the area first. The needle had a little camera on it so they could see me internally. I heard a click and felt a pinch as they took the sample. Then they maneuvered the needle around and took more samples. I am not even sure how many were taken.

We did the right breast first, the one that already had two recent surgical procedures. Then it began bleeding a lot. I had no idea why. (My later research suggests my DCIS may have created more blood vessels to allow the cancer to spread and grow.) Vicky applied pressure to my breast, yet I still acquired a hematoma, swollen blood clot, the size of a small fist. I now had a hard mass in my already bruised and cut up breast.

The doctor drew a pen mark around the hematoma and suggested I watch it. If it worsened then I must go to the emergency room that night. Vicky helped me fill my prescription of Vicodin for the pain. I was pretty upset about the whole procedure and was really cold and shaking. Vicky wrapped me in a blanket while I shivered, and walked me to Samantha's car. Thankfully, Samantha was there to drive me home. I could not have driven.

To pass along some advice, don't have a procedure that could become problematic late in the day or on a Friday. You want time to get back in to see a doctor if you need to.

I took the Vicodin for the pain forgetting how it had affected me in the past. I become wired instead of sleepy. I had my first panic attack and tossed in bed all night. I finally got out of bed and went over to the couch to watch TV. I checked my hematoma every few minutes convinced it had grown bigger and firmer. I didn't know what might happen if the hematoma worsened so my imagination began playing tricks with me. I kept the phone close to me in case I needed to call 911. I tried my best to go it alone, yet at 5:00 a.m. I woke up mom and Paul.

I felt my heart racing. It must be a heart attack, I thought. Paul hugged me while assuring me this was a panic attack. I scheduled an appointment with a doctor for an EKG and a chest X-ray. Afterward, they guaranteed me everything was fine. This helped yet the hematoma continued to worry me. This big hard mass in my breast lingered for several months. It was even there when I had the mastectomies though it had subsided a bit.

A few days later Dr. X called to share they found no more cancer in the tissue samples they removed in my stereotactic biopsies. Based on my mammogram and stereotactic biopsy results, she didn't think I needed an MRI. She also shared that the downtime after the mastectomies would be about four weeks. I told her I preferred to stay in the hospital over-night and would not have the surgery as an outpatient. She noted this and told me Dr. S would perform the post-operation follow-up. I also asked her for a prescription for the special camisole with little pockets for the surgical drains. She mentioned she'd write it for me.

I asked whether to take Xanax or Excedrin PM to help me sleep. She recommended the Excedrin PM. I also told her I thought I'd wait until September or October for the mastectomies due to our pre-paid trip to Italy on August 11th. She thought it would be fine to reschedule my surgery, and she'd be available in both September and October.

As I've mentioned earlier, I originally wanted the surgery sooner than July 10th. Since I needed the general surgeon to do the mastectomies and the reconstructive surgeon to start this process; this meant coordinating between their schedules. I also didn't feel comfortable leaving the country, or even flying, so soon after surgery. In retrospect this proved to be very smart decision. I would not have been physically or mentally ready for a physically demanding trip a month after my mastectomies.

Due to the hematoma, my positive results from the stereotactic biopsies, and my need for rest from having surgery, I rescheduled the mastectomies from July to September 5, 2006. When I made my decision to get the mastectomies, I wanted the surgery done as fast as possible. I didn't care to continue walking around with cancer, like some ticking time-bomb.

Rescheduling the mastectomies allowed us to finally go on our trip to Italy. We'd been planning it for years. We spent two weeks in Italy including three nights in Rome, four nights in Florence, and a week outside of Venice. We had a great time as a family, especially sharing this experience with our daughter, Gabby, the best traveler of our family. Each day, she prepared her backpack filling it with snacks, water, her camera, hat, and things to entertain herself with. It brought me so much joy to observe her enjoying everything so much.

All this said, I still think it would have been better for me to have postponed the trip and have the surgery over with. The upcoming surgery weighed on my mind like a piece of heavy luggage all through Italy and beyond. For the first time ever I needed to take Xanax for anxiety and/or to sleep, along with, Tylenol and Excedrin PM on a regular basis.

As I've shared before, the worst part of this whole breast cancer experience occurred between my diagnosis on May 10th and the mastectomies on September 5th. My mind was really a mess. I think the mental aspect of this whole thing weighed far worse than any physical issues. Overall I am grateful I took our special trip with my family because one never knows what can happen in surgery. If I had died, at least they would have the extraordinary memories from our trip.

The day scheduled for my surgery, September 5, 2006, happened to be Gabby's first day of fifth grade. It is challenging to schedule both surgeons on the same day, so I had to do it when they were both available. I had also longed to go to my 20 year college reunion in Chicago at the end of September. This wouldn't happen now. I couldn't put off the mastectomies any longer. There will always be a holiday or some event to interfere with taking care of major health issues. But health must come first, so I implore you to schedule your surgeries and appointments as soon as possible. Without our health, we have nothing.

THE DAYS BEFORE MY BILATERAL MASTECTOMIES

August 29, 2006

I had a pre-operation visit with Dr. X, seven days before my scheduled mastectomies. She was kind of aloof and hurried me. We didn't spend as much time talking as we had on other visits. I would have liked a little more compassion and empathy, especially from another woman. Perhaps being a surgeon she must remain emotionally detached from her patients.

POINTS FROM DR. BARRY:

- ### A surgeon is on a tight schedule.

Next I signed a consent form to have the bilateral mastectomies. I wondered why they were referring to my left breast removal as prophylactic. I sure didn't of it that way. It seemed necessary to me. The consent form said this procedure would not increase my chance of survival. I found this troublesome. Then why did I agree to have my boobs cut off? I thought this procedure would increase my chance of survival.

I had the nurse call Dr. X back so we could talk about this some more. She met with me in the hallway and said, "Yes, how can I help you?"

I wanted to say, "Lady you can help me by not cutting off my boobs. You can tell me this is a bad dream." Instead I asked, "Why am I having this procedure if it does not increase my chance of survival?"

She mumbled something about there not being enough studies or there was not enough data to indicate that "prophylactic mastectomies" increased survival rates. She then said, "Just have the surgery."

I still don't completely understand this. If problem is eliminated as best as possible by taking out tissue prone to breast cancer, why wouldn't this increase one's chance of survival through decreasing one's risk of getting breast cancer?

POINTS FROM DR. BARRY:

- **Although the above statement seems to be intuitive, you can't assume it to be true without scientific evidence.**
- **To date there is no scientific evidence to support this theory.**
- **It's the evidence based theories of Western Medicine, different from law which is arrived at by a bunch of opinions.**
- **Opinions can and do change with time and have little basis in fact. Science attempts to minimize opinion by forming a hypothesis (i.e. removing breast tissue eliminates breast cancer).**
- **Then you test the hypothesis, ideally with a randomized, double-blinded study (i.e. randomly assign a group of women to either have their breasts removed or not then choose another doctor-not involved-to follow them for development of breast cancer.) It attempts to eliminate the inherent bias of opinion.**

Based on the consent form and my brief conversation with Dr. X, I nearly cancelled my surgery. However, from what the oncologist, Dr. P, and my research indicated, if I did nothing, my risk of having a recurrence of breast cancer substantially increased. There would be a 50/50 chance it could return as invasive or non-invasive cancer. In some women the DCIS remains dormant. But in other women it will become invasive cancer. The challenge is no one knows in which women it will become full blown cancer or when it will happen. Basically, it is like walking around with a slow, ticking time bomb that might or might not explode.

I tried to be objective about a treatment choice, yet maybe after I found my answer, I didn't gather enough information on the others. Having young children, I don't want to live in fear of a recurrence. I would also prefer to not take medications with other side effects like increasing my risk for other cancers and/or ushering in my change of life prematurely. Being so afraid of the unknown, the thought of having a recurrence of breast cancer terrified me. I again focused on how I'd be getting the boobs of a 20-year-old; I'd view this as a "boob job." This was the only way for me to get through this.

Prior to surgery, on August 31, 2006, I met with Dr. S's physician assistant, Cindy, for a pre-op visit. She photographed my breasts and felt them. Cindy confirmed it best to remove my nipples, which seemed odd. We all have nipples. If no one else had them, it wouldn't matter. I really couldn't imagine how they would take my nipples and leave enough skin for a new breast. (Somehow they did leave me enough skin and my new breasts look great.)

POINTS FROM DR. BARRY:

- **It is common for patients to block out or forget what is said during a doctor's visit.**
- **Some people tape record their visits with the doctor.**

45

MY MASTECTOMIES

September 5, 2006

Paul and I took our daughter to school for her first day of fifth grade. I would normally never leave my house without make-up on, yet today I did. We settled Gabby in to her new class; then Paul told the teacher I had surgery scheduled so Gabby might have a difficult day. I knew if I spoke to the teacher, I'd do so with tears streaming down my face. I kissed my girl good-bye and prayed I'd see her again that night.

Paul drove me to the hospital for my skin-sparing (taking the breast tissue while leaving as much skin as possible to create a breast mound), bilateral (both breasts), mastectomies. I checked in with admissions right around 9:00 a.m. I had fasted since midnight and could only have water or clear fluids until 8:30 a.m. Since I normally eat an early breakfast, I felt famished. I sat in a small waiting room looking around at the other people in there. Of course, I first noticed a lady who had no hair. I hoped this wouldn't be a bad omen for me. Dr. X and Dr. P both told me, and my research also indicated if they didn't find anything more than DCIS (non-invasive cancer in my ducts), I would not need radiation, chemotherapy, or any other medications. I prayed to God to only have DCIS.

They called me in to a room in the nuclear medicine department and a friendly doctor injected radioactive dye into each breast. Paul kept me company during this procedure but looked away at the sight of needles. I still pondered backing out of the surgery to just take my chances. After all this upcoming surgery wasn't going to increase my chances of survival according to the release I signed through my insurance. Paul had preferred I live more vicariously and take my chances with what may happen by doing nothing, yet he still supported whatever decision I made.

The doctor explained the radioactive dye would travel to my lymph nodes, and then Dr. X could do a sentinel node biopsy. This meant she would only remove one or two lymph nodes, considered the main lymph nodes and the most likely to have cancer if it were to spread. If they found no cancer in these main lymph nodes then the surgeon wouldn't need to take out any more. I still had this huge urge to throw off my hospital gown, get dressed, and run as fast as I could out away from this hospital.

Sentinel node biopsies are relatively new procedures. Instead of taking out all of the lymph nodes under the armpit, a skilled surgeon can find and remove the first lymph node that cancer may have spread to. If this lymph node doesn't have cancer then there usually isn't a need to take out more lymph nodes. If it is positive for cancer then more lymph nodes will need to be removed. It is best to have only a few lymph nodes taken out if possible for healing purposes and to avoid lymphedema (swelling of the fingers, hands, and/or arms). I will explain mastectomies, lymphedema, sentinel node biopsy, and reconstruction in more detail later in this book.

When my grandmother had her mastectomy in the early 1980's, I don't think they did sentinel node biopsies. She had all or most of the lymph nodes under her armpit taken out. Mastectomies were more radical then. Her chest appeared concave where her breast had been, and it was not attractive to look at. She did not have reconstruction but wore a fake breast, prosthetic, in her bra. I remember how she would take it out and hand it to the men in the family for laughs. Fortunately, advances are underway in how a mastectomy is performed and also with the reconstruction process.

Returning to my surgery, the radioactive dye felt warm and tingly as it traveled through my system. I said another prayer for it only to be DCIS, and that I would live through the surgery eventually having nice, reconstructed 20-year-old breasts.

They brought me into another waiting area and then called me into surgery. After they began pumping me with drugs, I don't remember a thing until after they wheeled me to my room following four hours of surgery. Dr. X performed a sentinel node biopsy removing two lymph nodes from my right arm pit area and one lymph node from my left. She removed as much breast tissue as possible including my nipples and areolas while leaving as much of my skin intact as she could. Dr. S started the reconstruction process by putting muscle expanders, temporary implants, underneath my chest muscles.

The attendant wheeled me into my room. My room-mate had drawn the curtain so I didn't see her. Paul and my daughter, Gabby, came to visit me later in the day. She cried when she saw the IV hooked up to me. She climbed into bed with me, and I cuddled with her. Her need to be strong during this whole ordeal must have taken a lot out of her. I think she finally understood what had happened and needed to collapse. She seemed more herself after we snuggled and talked. Sometimes I can forget that my smart, brave girl is really just a little girl. She was only nine when I had my mastectomies.

My friend Lynn popped in for a few minutes; and my mom and my brother Jeffrey also came to visit. I felt drugged up and don't recall much about their visits. I had a catheter and could not get out of bed. I felt so weak. I looked down and noticed my chest all bandaged up. Thankfully, it did not look completely flat. I couldn't handle leaving the operating table with a totally flat chest.

That evening my nurse told me to rest and not to worry about my lack of energy. I couldn't even get out of bed. She would make sure the morning nurse helped me to get out of bed and to walk. I slept and still felt exhausted the next morning. The physical and mental trauma of the surgery wiped me out. If you have a mastectomy, I suggest you not go home that day. In my view, a mastectomy should not be done on an outpatient basis.

September 6, 2006

That morning, I watched TV, slept, and asked my nurse for help out of bed and to walk me around. She lifted me so I could dangle my feet over the bed and then mentioned she'd be back in a few minutes. She still hadn't returned 20 minutes later. She was nothing like my nurse the night before. I wondered if she'd ever come back.

The attendant who brought me to my room the day before rolled my room-mate in. I heard her moaning. The nurse came into the room, and they both tried to get my room-mate into her bed. Apparently she wasn't able to do what they were asking her to do. While they were working with her, the head nurse came in to talk with me. Thankfully, she heard the commotion behind the curtain. She walked over and began questioning the nurse and the patient. The patient could not respond to any of the questions the head nurse asked her. All I heard were loud groans. They called a "code blue"and within minutes 12-15 doctors and nurses showed up in our room.

Someone pushed my bed over to the side and into the wall. My feet were still over the side, and I felt trapped. I had a catheter and an IV attached to me and just didn't have the strength to get back into bed or to get out of the room. They were attempting to resuscitate my room-mate. I started shaking. I felt so alone.

Fortunately, a nurse recognized this. She asked, "Can you walk?"

I said, "No."

She said, "I'll be right back with a wheel chair."

She came over for me and wheeled me into the next room. My body still trembled. I had never experienced anything like this before.

About a half hour later the head nurse came to check on me. She found me sobbing and reached over to hug me. I learned my room-mate had a bad reaction to the anesthesia she had been given during surgery and had been moved to the intensive care department. They expected her to pull through, not sure if she did. I thanked the nurse for checking in on me because the other nurse probably would not have known what to do with my room-mate. She might have died in the other nurse's care. After this experience I couldn't wait to get out of the hospital.

The next nurse seemed far more attentive. She assisted me out of bed and helped me to the bathroom. My mom spent her 73rd birthday having dinner with me at the hospital. Now this is true love when someone is willing to eat hospital food for their birthday dinner. I could barely move and still had a catheter and an IV in. Mom walked me slowly around the nurses' station; kind of sad when my mother could walk faster and for longer than me.

Next my friend Tanya visited me. Then after she left Jocelyn came over. She told me about her high blood pressure. Ironically the nurse took my blood pressure about this same time, and it was high. Now I began to worry about high blood pressure. I may have driven up the numbers with my fears.

RECOVERY and RECONSTRUCTION

September 7, 2006

After two nights in the hospital, I returned home. Although weak I felt thrilled to be home. I slept on the coach and the recliner for a few nights because I couldn't make it up the stairs to my bedroom. Drains dangled out of each breast area, and I wore the special camisole with the little pouches to put the drains in. I didn't want to frighten anyone with bloody tubes hanging from me. My mom helped me empty the drains three or four times a day. There was a special way to open them, squeeze them, and then pour the contents into a measuring cup. We had to monitor how much bloody fluid came out of each breast and when we did the draining. If you go through this, make sure you have someone there with you. This was a disgusting and tedious experience I don't know how I would have done it without Mom. I didn't want Paul or Gabby to go through this with me. I had an On-Q device pumping pain medication directly into each breast. I really didn't feel much pain, maybe due to all my follow-up meds. Taking pain pills had me wired instead of sleepy but cut the pain, and antibiotics helped prevent an infection.

When Mom first looked at my breast area about a week after my mastectomies, she started crying. She told me it wasn't because it looked bad. It broke her heart to see me go through all of this. I couldn't even look at my chest in the mirror or at all.

I also couldn't shower for the first week, so I took sponge baths, and my mom washed my hair for me in the sink. It seemed like camping except in my own home. As I've mentioned, I could not have managed without my mother during this time. I wear contacts or glasses because I am nearsighted. Not having the best vision worked well. I just kind of blurred my vision and didn't look straight down at my breast area.

The next day Paul's sister, Pauline, drove me to see Dr. S, the reconstructive surgeon. When I told Dr. S and the nurses I couldn't look at myself Dr. S said , "That is fine, I'm your eyes."

Dr. S also shared that everything looked "great." I didn't know if our versions of "looking great" were in sync. Yet he checked my surgical sites and assured me that I was healing nicely.

During the surgery they removed and analyzed three lymph nodes, two from my problematic right side and one from my left side. On September 12, 2006 Dr. X called to tell me my lymph nodes had been fully analyzed, and there was no sign of cancer. I felt this huge relief ripple through me like a wave passing across the ocean. If they had found cancer, I would have needed another surgery to remove more lymph nodes, along with courses of chemotherapy and/ or radiation.

The pathologist also analyzed my breast tissue. My left breast was benign meaning they did not find any breast cancer. My right breast, however, had 2.5 cm (about an inch) of high grade DCIS. All margins were cancer free, and they found no evidence of invasive cancer. Based on these results Dr. X shared there was nothing more for me to do. I would not need Tamoxifen, radiation, or chemotherapy. I felt so liberated. Yeah!

What continued to disturb me though is that I still had about an inch (2.5 cm) of cancer that had gone undetected. As you may recall, I had an ultrasound, mammograms, a needle biopsy, physical examinations, two surgical biopsies, acupuncture, and stereotactic biopsies to examine the most suspicious areas in my breasts. None of these screening devices or biopsies picked up the additional inch of cancer.

The DCIS taken out in my original biopsies were 3 mm (about half the size of a pencil eraser) and 1.6 mm (about a quarter of a pencil eraser) in size. Yet an inch of early stage cancer lurked in my breast. I am so grateful I had the mastectomies to remove cancer which may have gone undetected for years. Who knows what could have happened in the future.

All things considered, I had a fairly easy recovery. On September 15th, Pauline drove me to Dr. S's office; and I finally had those revolting drains taken out. Nurse Barbara removed the major bandages and padding from my chest. With all of this padding, I felt like a football player. It had constricted my breathing. I also couldn't lift my arms very high, but every day my movement improved. I could move my left arm easier than my right arm. I asked Dr. S if I needed physical therapy, but he didn't think so. He recommended I apply antiseptic to the area where the drains came out of my skin and on the scars. My mom did this for me a few times a day. Dr. S said I could now wear sports bras for some support and that hopefully, the next week we'd begin my saline injections to expand my new breast mounds. He also congratulated me on the pathology results - only DCIS.

I still found my recovery to be challenging on some levels. Even cutting a bagel seemed like a major work out. I could sure feel the muscles that were being used for that minor sawing motion and it hurt. Shutting a window, an activity I wouldn't have given another thought to, created pain. Lifting my arm to pull the cord to turn on the light in my garage became another challenge, along with shutting the trunk of my SUV. Tasks I had never given thought to now brought on stiffness and pain. Eventually all of these movements became easier as my range of motion in my arms improved.

For the first few weeks I didn't experience too much pain. However, as my feeling came back, the pain increased. I had no feeling when my mom touched me to put the antibiotic ointment on my scars. It seemed like my breasts and skin had frozen. Over time my nerves, skin, and muscles regained their sensitivity. With that I still have some minor pain. (I am happy to share that three years after my mastectomies, I have full movement in my arms. I'm also physically stronger and more muscular than I have been in my entire life, partly because I aggressively worked out with a young, handsome personal trainer for the last eighteen months. He pushes me to do arm and chest exercises I thought I could never do. I also ran my first half marathon (13.1 miles) without stopping or walking, in January of 2010. Having never been a runner, this was a major accomplishment for me.)

September 16, 2006

I celebrated my 42nd birthday and was thankful to be alive. Paul made his delightful enchiladas and surprised me with a decadent chocolate birthday cake. I enjoyed being surrounded with my family and a few friends for my birthday yet it also felt kind of exhausting to have a lot of people and so much noise in my home only 11 days after my surgery. I now understood how my grandma felt when she complained about the noise during big family gatherings.

Two weeks after my surgery, I could drive around the neighborhood if necessary. Seventeen days afterward Paul's Aunt Jill drove me to my appointment with Dr. S. since I wasn't ready to drive on the freeway yet. I still felt somewhat lightheaded after the procedures with Dr. S.) He checked my progress and gave me my first saline injection to expand my temporary implants. I hadn't even looked at my breast areas yet. I thought the procedure might cause pain or limited movement which I didn't want to interfere with a wedding I planned to attend the next day. Dr. S assured me I'd be fine. Fortunately, he was right

I had this procedure four times over the course of the next six weeks. Each procedure took about 10 minutes. I looked away as Dr. S did the work so I don't know exactly what happened. I know he numbed the area with a shot of some kind, he waited a few minutes and injected a specific amount of saline into a valve in both of my temporary implants. The reason for using the temporary implants, muscle expanders, is to allow in more saline over a period of time, thus, stretching the muscles and skin to prepare for the placement of permanent implants. I wish someone would invent a permanent implant that could be expanded, thus, alleviating the need for another surgery to replace the temporary one.

POINTS FROM DR. BARRY:

- **According to Dr. Barry, there is such an implant. See www.mentorcorp.com and look for "siltex spectrum" implants regarding temporary implants that can be permanent implants.**

September 22, 2006

I still had a limited range of motion in my arms, and I began to fear my movement wouldn't return. I went on the internet to research the right exercises to do after a mastectomy. See http://www.cancer.org/docroot/CRI/content/CRI_2_6x_Exercises_After_Breast_Surgery.asp (those are underscores after CRI 2 6x Exercises After Breast). The site offers exercises that can be done after a breast biopsy, lymph node removal, lumpectomy, mastectomy, or breast reconstruction. The site also recommends checking with your doctor prior to beginning the exercises so I printed out all six pages of exercises to show Dr. S and Nurse Barbara. Please check with your doctor before you start exercising.

Dr. S said the exercises would be fine, and he also approved my doing yoga again when I felt ready. Nurse Barbara shared that she had breast cancer about 15 years before and went through radiation. Somehow it froze her arm, and she needed physical therapy to regain her movement.

We discussed nutrition, and she recommended a diet higher in omega-3 acids, with flaxseed oil, lots of green vegetables, and cabbage. She also recommended a strong multivitamin. (I now take Usana supplements. You can contact me if you would like to try them.) We need to boost our immune systems throughout our lives, yet if we are at a higher risk for cancer, or have been diagnosed with cancer, it is even more critical to do so.

Exercising, practicing yoga, lifting small weights, and doing some machines at the gym helped me, and I did not need physical therapy.

Eventually I no longer felt pain cutting a bagel, shutting a window, pushing a grocery cart, shutting the trunk on my SUV, combing my hair, pulling on a shirt, or reaching overhead to pull a light cord. However, it took months to gradually increase my movement and flexibility.

After surgery, don't push yourself too much and don't do anything which feels painful. Do attempt to regain your normal life and normal movements as soon as your body allows it. Listen to your own body and definitely check with your doctor about what you can and cannot do.

Keeping my gym membership active proved to be a smart idea. (I began working out at 18-years-old.) There were a few weeks here or there when I didn't make it to the gym, yet I exercised fairly often. I wanted to return to the gym as soon as possible after every procedure. I enjoyed seeing familiar faces and getting back into my routine. Each time I did whatever I could and then felt pleased with myself as I progressed. None of my gym acquaintances knew about my breast cancer. The gym became a safe haven for me.

I had my first big night out. Paul's niece, Sarah, hosted her rehearsal dinner at her home. Only thing is I barely remember it. My continued use of pain medication had worn me out. We went to her wedding the next day. I still hadn't seen my breast area, yet I managed to get dressed up. I couldn't lift a top over my head so I had to step into my top and pull it up. I surprised myself by dancing through a song or two with my daughter Gabby and my sister-in-law Janie.

Even though it may not seem like it, I thought I was in a good place. I had accepted the mastectomies yet didn't want to risk freaking myself out by looking at my breast area. I wanted to heal first and have Dr. S expand my new breasts before I saw them. I couldn't imagine what I would look like with a nipple-less scarred breast. Avoiding them worked for me. I wore a sports bra that zipped up in the front and another one which had hooks in the front. I could do both by slightly peering down but without noticing my breasts. I wore my old silk shirts that buttoned up, were loose fitting, and left over from my days as an attorney. I did start looking at myself in the mirror while wearing a sports bra, just not naked. I began to like the shape I saw in the mirror. It was as if I'd become a teenager developing again. Every time I saw Dr. S, I increased my size a little more. Dr. S and his nurses Barbara and Robyn were so kind to me. Along with my breasts, we also developed friendship.

During one of my visits to Dr. S's office, the nurse took my blood pressure on my thigh so I could avoid lymphedema. (See my section on lymphedema and avoiding lymphedema.) I found out my blood pressure was very high. The nurse told me to contact my regular doctor. Given this happened on a Friday, I didn't hear back from anyone until Monday. I rested on the couch during the weekend, convinced I'd caused myself a new problem, high blood pressure. It turned out later to be fine. I learned a blood pressure reading from your thigh gives a much higher reading than a reading from your arm. Many nurses don't know how to take blood pressure on the thigh. They need to use a special thigh cuff, not a regular cuff for the arm.

Overall, I began focusing more on what I have: my life, family, friends, people I care about and who care about me, than what I lost, my breasts. In the bigger life picture losing my breasts is not that big of a deal. Although I must admit, I am a vain woman. Soon after my mastectomies I placed more attention on my other positive physical attributes. I have beautiful eyes, great legs, and a shapely body. Now a few years afterward, I think my breasts look even better than they did before the mastectomies.

My breasts served their purpose, they breastfed two children. They were perky B cups earlier on, but after two kids and turning 40 they became a bit saggy. I wouldn't have undergone a boob job, mainly because I think it would be challenging to find breast cancer with implants. Having breast cancer again slightly worries me now. Since I lowered my risk to 0-2%, this is a level I'm comfortable with. Given my vanity which I believe many of us women share, I could not have had the mastectomies if it meant leaving the table with no breasts. The implants were a necessity for me even though I've never been into cosmetic surgery.

These new breasts are mine. It is my skin, just not my tissue. I still have my muscle but a silicon shell, replaced my cancerous tissue. So which door will I choose? Cancerous tissue or noncancerous fake boobs? I'll take door number 2. I thank God and all of my health care providers, family and friends, for all they did to help me get through this experience.

September 29, 2006

I visited Dr. S. This time I drove myself. His office is about 20 miles from my house via the freeway. I used the small pillow given to me by the breast coordinator after my mastectomies. Another breast cancer survivor made it. It kept the seatbelt from rubbing against my incisions. I still had not seen my new, naked breast. I had noticed that the right side under my arm pit was indented more than the left side from looking at my breasts with my sports bra covering them. Dr. S explained this was left over from my previous biopsies and that it might not fill in. I also noticed the scars were thicker than when I had the biopsies. He said they'd fade over time. Then I wondered why the veins in my hands seemed more pronounced. Again, Dr. S put me at ease.

I think I had become too hyper-vigilant about everything that seemed the least bit strange. I may have lost some trust and confidence in my own body and well-being by going through this major medical event.

Next I had another injection of saline into my muscle expander, temporary implants. Dr. S told me he put in 100 c.c's of saline in each breast in the operating room during reconstruction. He applied 60 c.c's on September 23rd and another 60 cc's on this visit. Thus, I had 220 cc's of saline in each implant, and he would fill them to 350 ccs. So, I was about 2/3 full.

October 3, 2006

I returned to my yoga class. I could do most of the moves. This felt energizing. I did not lift my arms fully above my head or do down dog (an inverted "v"). I mostly did legs and balance work. I modified what I had to and just did what felt right for my body.

I share this because I was not going to let breast cancer or my surgeries get in the way of my life. It felt so important to get my life back. I would recommend you do the same if you are in a similar situation. Every day I got mentally and physically stronger. You will too!

October 6, 2006

I drove myself to Dr. S's office for another injection of saline, thus bigger breasts. I could now observe myself in the mirror with a bra on more frequently and could even pull the bra down to look at the top part of my breast. It was still my skin. I had those familiar little dots I've always had. I started pulling the bra up to see the lower portion of my breast. It seemed nice and round, but I still had indents under the breast area and on the sides. I didn't see myself as a whole. I avoided the scars. Only my mother, doctors and nurses, had seen my naked breasts so far.

I next asked Dr. S if I could do gardening. He okayed it if I wore gloves. Since my surgery on September 5th, I couldn't lift my almost two-year-old, Andrew. This was very difficult for both of us. I had nursed him until May and now couldn't hold him. I sat down first and then let him climb into my lap. We still cuddled but someone else had to pick him up to place him in his bathtub or his crib. Then someone else had to take him out of his bath or crib. Interesting how I had done all these things before without a thought. Finally, on this day, in addition to gardening, I had the doctor's approval to lift Andrew again. As a bonus, I could even lift small weights at the gym.

Before the mastectomies I slept on my side, yet with surgery on both breasts, both sides caused me pain. Afterward I slept almost in a sitting position propped up by many pillows. Dr. S said I could sleep on my side. He also told me my breasts would fill in more with permanent implants. He recommended I improve my physical condition as much as possible before the next surgery to put in my permanent implants for an easier recovery.

I mentioned my blood pressure experience to Dr. S from the week before. I wondered why the nurse who took my blood pressure didn't know that a woman who has had a mastectomy should have her blood pressure done on the other arm. In my case, having had had both breasts removed, I'm supposed to have blood pressure taken on the thigh. Since these nurses deal with patients with mastectomies on a regular basis, they need to know what to do. He said he would talk to the nurses. I thought this might improve the experience for the next woman in my situation.

Although I may have been over cautious I feared developing lymphedema. (Something I had never heard of until after my breast cancer diagnosis. Lymphedema is the temporary or permanent swelling of the hand, arms and/or fingers.) I avoided heavy lifting, exposure to dirt when gardening, and took care not to get cuts on my hands and arms. I didn't use a regular razor to shave under my arms. Instead I used a small battery-operated one which doesn't have a blade. I also took my blood pressure on my thigh.

I found it important to socialize and to be as active as possible. I participated in business meetings, lunches with friends, and yoga classes. I worked when I could and listened to my body. I gave myself the six weeks of time a woman needs after having a baby to recuperate. Six weeks after my surgery, I hosted my daughter Gabby's 10th birthday party at our home. Fortunately, we plan most things in advance, so we already had all of the supplies for her craft project, along with her party favors.

A week later I even wore a two piece bathing suit to a business mixer at a day spa. I put it on in a small changing area. I didn't want anyone to see me, especially since I hadn't looked at myself yet. Yet I acknowledged myself for taking another bold step.

October 20, 2006

I went in for another injection of saline with Dr. S. This time I could immediately see the results, bigger breasts. I mentioned the pain I experienced when lying on my sides. He said the discomfort was normal, it meant my senses in that area were returning. We discussed my upcoming surgery for my permanent implants. According to Dr. S, recovery would be much smoother than after the mastectomies.

I would not likely need drains; however, he would put in the pain relieving On-Q pump to manage any soreness. He stressed it would be very important to limit my lifting and movement after this surgery because he wanted the implants to settle in right.

October 26, 2006

I did as much "normal" stuff as I could before the next surgery, and every day I felt stronger and better. Although I'm still not sure I could completely face what I had been through. I didn't look at my breast area until October 26th, about seven weeks after my mastectomies. While getting ready to meet my friend, Carol, for lunch, I walked over to the mirror and looked. Until then as I've mentioned, I would avoid seeing them as I dressed, while in the shower and, especially, in front of mirrors. Actually, with each new injection from Dr. S I noticed more of a breast mound. As I've mentioned before, I would lift my bra up a bit and look at the lower part of my breast area or pull my bra down and look at the top part. But, until now, I hadn't seen the whole area.

When I finally took a look at myself in the mirror, I smiled. The scars weren't too bad, I had my own skin, and the breasts were perky mounds. I missed my nipples though. Yet, overall, the experience turned out much better than I'd thought.

November 5, 2006

With my increasing strength, two months after my mastectomies, I walked the Susan G. Komen Race for the Cure in Balboa Park. I have participated other times, but this time it hit home. I walked as a breast cancer "survivor." The good and the bad news is I am definitely not alone. There were thousands of people at the event, many wearing pink caps, shirts and/or feather boas. Most of the survivors looked great, yet some did not look too healthy. I cried a little during the opening ceremonies, when I looked around and took in all of the "survivors." This disease hits women of all ages, heights, weights, colors, and ethnicities. We must find a cure for breast cancer!

The race is a 5 kilometer (3.1 mile) walk or run. My daughter Gabby and my friends Carolyn, Jocelyn, Tanya, and their daughters

Lauren and Cara did it with me. Mom drove over with us but stayed at the starting area. She didn't think she could walk the hills. I appreciated the support and companionship of these special women in my life – the young and the old.

I wasn't sure I'd finish it since I hadn't regained my full strength, but I completed it without having to sit and rest. I wanted to give myself a high five. There were some strenuous areas where we had to go up or down hill, yet we had a beautiful San Diego day to encourage us along. We all finished the walk through Balboa Park and over closed highways without a problem. After the walk we went back to the "survivors" tent and I received a small gift bag with some moisturizers and a pink carnation. I also had a free 10 minute back massage. Now that felt great.

I realized during the walk, and then contemplated it more afterward, that having breast cancer or being a "survivor" is not my identity. It is only something I experienced. I chose to have bilateral mastectomies to be proactive instead of feeling like a victim, waiting for something worse to happen.

November 13, 2006

I met with reconstruction surgeon, Dr. S for my final injection of saline. He told me he would fill me beyond capacity to stretch my muscles and skin to give me better results with my permanent implants. For a few days after each injection I ached since my muscles were stretching. I felt as if I'd just finished a strenuous workout.

I must reiterate that Dr. S was a godsend. He made my whole experience as bearable as possible. I even looked forward to our visits and chats. Selecting the right health provider is so important. We put our health, essentially our lives into their hands. Choose well.

November of 2006

I worked, attended networking lunches, got flu shots, and had my relatives over for dinner to celebrate Andrew's 2nd birthday. We played a lot too. We visited Legoland (a fun amusement park where many things are made out of Legos); watched the taping of the Hannah

61

Montana shows in Los Angeles; saw a musical; and the Mother Goose Parade. My life felt back to normal. Busy as ever.

I could finally drive without restrictions. What a relief. I still used a little pillow under my seat belt so that it wouldn't hit me rub against my surgical site. During Thanksgiving break, I drove mom, Gabby and Andrew to an old western town called Julian. It is a 90-minute drive through some windy roads and mountains. We had fun walking around, having lunch and going on a horse and carriage ride. Julian had been a gold rush town in the 1800's, and is now a charming, little town for tourists. Of course, we had some apple pie, one of the things Julian is famous for.

I spent the holidays with my family and it felt even more special this year. I secretly prayed to God for these not to be my last holidays. In spite of how well I'd been recovering, I dreaded my upcoming surgery. I have a deep fear that I will not wake up from anesthesia. To distract myself, I stayed busy and, whenever necessary, I took half of a Xanax pill for anxiety.

November 27, 2006

I saw a doctor because my heart started racing, and I worried about high blood pressure. He spent a lot of time talking to me reminding me to be good to myself. He said sometimes we are too hard on ourselves. It is normal to feel our bodies may have failed us by getting cancer or some other illness. We need to move on and not worry about our bodies so much. I felt a lot better.

December of 2006

Paul and I took the kids to Disneyland. I drove the two hours or so each way and seemed fine. I had my energy back and felt almost fully recovered. I just had some pain on the sides of my chest. During the night I woke up feeling stiff, and in the morning I would wake up with a very taut chest.

As always, the time between Thanksgiving and Christmas seemed a blur with activities, functions and parties. In mid-December my sister-in-law Pauline had her yearly tea in memory of her friend Sue, who died from breast cancer. I told her guests my story, and they were all very supportive and interested in my experience. Unfortunately, everyone knows someone who has had breast cancer.

A word of advice, be careful what you share with people who have breast cancer. I wanted to hear the positive stories about the women who had breast cancer and went on with their lives. I really didn't want to hear about the women who died or were diagnosed with other types of cancers. Think about this. If you get breast cancer, you can survive and lead a normal life. Your life can be as you knew it, or perhaps even better with your new perspective. Do not share horror stories about treatment nightmares, and the dreadful things so and so went through, with someone who shares he/she has cancer. We do not want to hear it. I have enough of an imagination as it is. Plus I've heard enough and read enough to not want to hear anymore really sad stories.

December 21, 2006

I had a pre-operation appointment to discuss the installation of my permanent implants with Dr. S's physician assistant, Cindy. Gabby was home on winter break and wanted to go with me to my appointment. She still had not seen me without a bra. In the examining room, I said, "Gabby please turn away when Cindy examines me."

"Why, Mom?" Gabby asked.

"Would you find it strange to see a woman without nipples?" I asked her.

Gabby said "You don't have nipples, Mom?"

"Are you sure you wouldn't find it strange to see a woman without nipples?" I asked her again.

"It would be okay," she said.

"I don't have nipples." I bit my lip so as not to cry.

She said she wanted to see, so I pulled my gown open to show her. She stared for a moment and then said, "It looks better than I thought it would."

Who knows what this little girl thought I would look like? I couldn't even glance at myself for about seven weeks since I felt so afraid of what I might discover. Gabby's response and her strength brought a big smile to my face.

To return to the meeting with Cindy, I expressed my concern to her that one of my breasts appeared a little lower than the other. She told me Dr. S would do his best to correct this when he put in my permanent implants. I asked some questions about what to expect. She told me the surgery would take about two hours, and I'd go home with a medical bag with tubes which would feed pain medication directly into my breasts. (I also used these after my mastectomies. It is called OnQ and you can learn more about it at www.AskYourSurgeon.com.) Fortunately I would likely not have those disgusting drains coming out of me as I did with the mastectomies. Cindy also told me to limit my movement again meaning no lifting over five pounds. This also meant I wouldn't be able to lift my two-year-old son again, along with no major stretching of my arms for 6-8 weeks. I could drive again in about two weeks, though she stressed that I limit my movement more now than when I had the mastectomies. Dr. S didn't want my new implants to move around. Cindy told me it would be fine to take Tums for my acid reflux and Xanax for anxiety or problems sleeping in anticipation of the surgery. She also gave me a prescription of Percocet for pain after the surgery and for Keflex to fight any infections. She gave me her phone number and told me to call her if I had any more questions or concerns. I found Cindy to be a top-notch medical professional. Her extremely kind, caring, and knowledgeable ways put me at ease.

By the time of my surgery to have my temporary implants replaced with my permanent implants, my life had returned to normal. I had my own business as a mortgage broker and did most of my work from home via computer and telephone. About two weeks after my mastectomies, I started working a few hours a day. In October and November I began working more and increased my life's activities overall. I had a client who called me about two to five times a day in October and November. He didn't know about my recent cancer or surgery. I chose not to tell new clients about my situation. I didn't want them to think I couldn't get the job done for them. My client, David, helped me get me back on the work path even though he didn't know it. He became a great distraction for me.

PERMANENT IMPLANTS

December 26, 2006

I woke up at 4:00 a.m. on the morning of my surgery. The alarm had been set for 6:00 a.m. I took a shower and got ready to go. I prayed to God that I'd survive the surgery. Paul drove me to the hospital, and we arrived there around 7:00 a.m. My surgery would begin at 9:30 a.m. I don't know what I had been thinking when I scheduled this on the day after Christmas. I missed all of the good sales.

Dr. S and his assistant, Cindy, spoke with me while I waited in the hospital bed. Dr. S assured me he would do all he could to give me even, beautiful new breasts and that I'd get through the surgery just fine. The anesthesiologist came in to talk with me. I once again explained my fear of not waking up and asked for just enough anesthesia to keep me asleep during the procedure because I preferred to wake up right after the procedure. She said she would do her best. (The memories of my hospital room-mate having a bad reaction to her anesthesia still haunted me.) I remember nothing after that. Not even if Paul said good bye and/or kissed me or being wheeled to surgery or anything about the surgery.

What I believe happened with the surgery was Dr. S opened me up, took out the temporary implants/muscle expanders, put in my new implants and closed me up again. There could easily be more to it than that, but I didn't care to know all of the details.

After a few hours of surgery, I do recall waking up in the post-op recovery room with a cheerful, male nurse taking me over to a second recovery room. The new nurse introduced himself as Len. I took that as a good sign because my deceased father's name is Leonard. I spent a few hours in recovery.

I returned home at about three in the afternoon and continued resting. I had no desire to stay in the hospital after this surgery. It wasn't as major as the mastectomies. Since I didn't get much rest in the hospital and after my code blue room-mate experience, I decided I'd be better off recovering at home.

At home, I bled more than expected. Some blood seeped through my gauze. I did not have drains but did have the drip of On-Q to alleviate the pain. I experienced some pain, yet overall I felt pretty good. I felt tempted to overdue it, but I remembered Dr. S telling me how important it would be to take it easy for 8 weeks so as not to move the implants.

December 27, 2006

I couldn't sleep. I woke up at 2:20 a.m. and began scribbling out an outline for this book. Pain pills seem to have the opposite effect on me. Instead of being in a deep sleep, I felt wide awake. I wrote 25 pages of messy notes for four hours.

January 23, 2007

I met with Dr. S so he could check on my implants. He said everything looked great, and I could resume all of my normal activities, such as, yoga, lifting weights and most importantly, picking up my son, Andrew again. He suggested I wear a bra for support and comfort. I learned they'd begin creating my nipples in about six to eight weeks during two office visits, about an hour for each one. He would use a local anesthetic, and someone would need to drive me. The nipples would be developed by using my scars. I had no idea how they would do this, yet I trusted Dr. S to give me the best nipples possible. About three weeks after the nipple creation, I'd return to have the areola portion tattooed on.

I wasn't in a rush to have my nipples created. I even considered not getting them at all. I liked the smooth look of not having a nipple sticking through my shirt, especially since I often went braless. I also felt like having a break from all of these procedures. I decided to wait until May, and meanwhile, contemplated not getting an actual nipple and, instead, getting flowers or butterflies tattooed on in place of the areolas (the area around the nipple).

May 10, 2007

The one year anniversary of my breast cancer diagnosis. I had received a call the day before from Dr. S's nurse, Barbara, for my permission to give out my number to another patient. I had offered to speak to women who would like more information. Interestingly enough their patient, Debbie, phoned me on this significant day. Debbie was 50 years old, and had been diagnosed with DCIS one week before. She had taken the gene testing and through this discovered she has the BRCA1 gene mutation which makes it more likely she will have breast cancer. (See my discussion about the gene mutation.) She had been considering a bilateral mastectomy and wanted to ask me some questions as well as see my new breasts. She came to my home, and we chatted for about an hour. I answered her questions, mainly about my recovery after each procedure. I also let her take a look at my breasts and also, feel them. She seemed a bit giddy. I figured she must be happy with my results. Just so you know, my new breasts do look great, especially in clothing. They look fine without clothes, but my scars are still visible. Now my new breasts are hard to the touch, resembling a softball, though somewhat softer. They don't feel like real breasts. The next day, I would begin the reconstruction of my nipples. I mentioned to Debbie that if no one else had nipples, I wouldn't bother getting them. I liked the smooth look under my tops. Nonetheless I ended up choosing the complete reconstruction job.

May 11, 2007

My friend, Tanya, drove me over to Dr. S's office, and he began creating my nipples. Mom had gone on a cruise with my brother Jeffrey to celebrate his 50th birthday. So Tanya babysat for Andrew during my procedure. They played legos in the waiting room, walked to Target, ate chocolate (didn't save me any), and visited the pet store. Andrew didn't even miss me and in future visits there asked if he could go to see the animals and have chocolate.

I don't recall when I first learned they would be taking off my nipples. I'd heard early on one can get cancer in the nipples, so when having a mastectomy the doctors recommend removing the nipples, along with as much breast tissue and cells as possible. Somehow this information didn't register with me until right before my mastectomies. Nipple removal still seems like such an odd concept to me.

The nipple reconstruction took place in a small surgery room at Dr. S's office. It took about 1.5 hours. He took some measurements from my collarbone to the center of my breasts and then across the breasts. He placed little white stickers shaped like nipples on my breasts.

I went into the bathroom, looked in a mirror, and adjusted the stickers to make them level yet centered on each breast mound. (I joked with Dr. S that he needs a laser level.) I stayed awake during the procedure. Dr. S injected each breast with something to freeze them and used part of my previous scars and skin to create the tips of nipples. It seemed like he twisted my skin around and around and also, covered my eyes with a small towel, so I couldn't watch him. We talked during the whole procedure about gardening, travel, politics and whatever topics came to mind and discovered we have many similar viewpoints.

Dr. S trimmed down the right nipple because he thought it was too big. I didn't want to know what that entailed. I looked down when he finished, and my new nipples appeared large and pointy. He said they would shrink some. I didn't want them to protrude too much. I actually liked the flatness of no nipple but wanted to get the finished product. After Nurse Barbara bandaged me up, my friend, Tanya, took me home and I felt ready to collapse. My anxiety had crept in for about 10 days before this procedure. Again, my fear of the unknown. My racing heart awakened me a many times during the night the week or so before this procedure. During the days I stayed busy, yet whenever I paused to think about it, my heart seemed to pound a faster than normal.

After my nipple construction, I still felt physically exhausted the next day, so I rested and read most of the day. I'd planned on going to my brother's 50th birthday party that night, about 45 miles from my home. I could have driven but I didn't want to push myself, so my niece's husband, Dave, picked us up and then drove us home. He drove 180 miles round trip to do this for me, a nice gesture. I felt better once I arrived at the party. The next day my right arm felt stiff, and I couldn't lift it overhead.

May 14, 2007

My left side now felt fine but the right side had become difficult to move. I didn't want to push it. I gave myself time to heal. I drove with a little pillow under my seatbelt so it wouldn't rub against my breasts. During all of my procedures, the left side healed first, and then the right side followed a few days later. Thinking each time I may not get all of my movement back or heal properly, frightened me now and then. Thankfully all went well overall. At first the little nipples turned out to be a bit crusty and bled a little, like a scraped knee. I could shower the day after the procedure and only had to put antibiotic ointment on the area and keep it covered with gauze.

A few weeks after the nipple procedure, I went to Dr. "N" (I later referred to her "N" to stand for nasty) because my heart began palpitating again. I had never seen this physician before. She didn't have very good bed side manners and yelled at me when I mentioned I eat chocolate every day. I will not compromise with chocolate. She ordered an EKG and it came back fine. I'm sure it had been related to my stress. Do not be surprised if your heart races, a version of panic attacks, or other strange symptoms after a breast cancer diagnosis or during your treatments. This happens often.

My blood pressure also seemed a bit high, or so I thought. I used to be about 110/70. I had the nurses take my blood pressure on my thigh to avoid lymphedema, so that was probably giving me a higher reading, but no one told me that the thigh reading measures higher than the arm. So, I continued thinking I had high blood pressure until I figured it out. If you have a single mastectomy, then you should have blood pressure, blood draws and shots on the unaffected side. Since I don't have a good side, I chose to get these things done on my thigh or elsewhere, but not in my arms.

POINTS FROM DR. BARRY:

- **Having blood drawn or blood pressure taken won't cause lymphedema.**
- **The rationale for not taking blood pressure or starting IV's or blood draws on the side that has had a mastectomy, lymph nodes removed, or radiation is to decrease the risk of infection in the limb that has lymphedema.**
- **Node dissection and radiation or clogging with metastases may contribute to lymphedema.**
- **Lymphedema is caused by a disruption of lymphatics to the limb either by removing the lymph node they drain to or by destroying them with radiation or clogging them with metastatic cancer.**

If you have a sentinel node biopsy, and they only take one or two lymph nodes, then your risk of getting lymphedema (swelling of the arms, hands, and/or fingers that may be permanent) is small as compared to a full axillary dissection where they take a lot of your lymph nodes from your armpit area. Whenever you have any lymph nodes removed, take precautions to avoid lymphedema. The more lymph nodes removed - the more caution that needs to be taken. (See my discussion of lymphedema on page 190.)

My friend Connie has lymphedema from her node dissection and radiation. Her hand and arm swell up like a balloon, and she must wear a special tight-fitting arm and hand glove/sleeve to help with it. To decrease your risk of lymphedema, you also need to avoid sunburn to the arms along with carrying heavy purses or other items on the affected side

It took a few months for my new nipples to ease up. For a month or so I looked like Farrah Fawcett in that famous poster of her with her nipples sticking out. (A year later the left nipple became flat, and the right nipple raised a tiny bit, ideal for me since I don't wear a bra. In retrospect, I would have been fine with skipping the nipple creation and just getting the tattoos.)

June 8, 2007

While at Dr. S's office to have my areolas tattooed, his nurse, Barbara, played around with little tubes of paint to choose the best combination of for my skin tone. It seemed like mixing make-up. Dr. S came in a few times, and we'd show him our selections. We finally agreed on the right color. I layed on the table while Dr. S froze the area, put two round stamp marks on each breast and then tattooed them in. We chatted for the hour or so that it took him to tattoo the areolas. He then placed small bandages on me which he said I could remove the next day. Paul picked me up and took me home. I noticed that my breasts had started bleeding through the bandage. I didn't know what to expect since I'd never had a tattoo. Fortunately it became scabby, so I put antiseptic on it, and the area healed well.

It took 13 months from my diagnosis of breast cancer to the completion of my new breasts. During this time I had bouts of crying and also, feeling angry that I had breast cancer yet, for the most part, I made my life as normal as possible. For me, the biggest challenge had been not knowing what to expect, between May and September of 2006. The surgeries weren't fun, but they could have been a lot worse. Most of all, I am so thankful I caught my breast cancer at such an early stage. You really must follow your instincts and be your own advocate. If I had stopped after the needle biopsy, the doctor's exam, the ultrasound, or the acupuncturist, I wouldn't have found the cancer. I listened to my instinct to have a biopsy so I would definitely know what was going on in my breast. Of course, I didn't expect to learn I had breast cancer. I felt certain the doctor would call to tell me she found scar tissue.

Late July, 2007

I now began to worry about ovarian cancer. The ladies in my bunco group mentioned a friend of theirs had died of ovarian cancer.

One of her symptoms had been bloating in the abdomen. Since my stomach had become proportionally bigger than the rest of me, I wondered now if there was a connection. I had read somewhere that stress causes more fat cells to store in your stomach. When a man I didn't know asked me if this was my first child, and a woman I had just met asked me about my due date, I felt more concerned about my fat tummy. I guess I should be flattered that at 42 years old, I looked young enough to still be thought of as pregnant and not just fat.

July 30, 2007

I visited my ob-gyn on who understood my concerns after having had breast cancer. He performed an ultrasound in the office and mentioned that my ovaries looked normal with no sign of cancer. I learned there is not a good test for detecting ovarian cancer. The CA125 test is not very accurate. He shared that a woman can be cancer free yet in three months have full-blown ovarian cancer. I told him I had already considered having the BRCA gene marker test to see if I had the gene mutation which increases the risk for breast and ovarian cancer. He recommended I have the test and ordered it for me. None of my other doctors had encouraged this procedure which surprised me.

August 2, 2007

Next a small area on my nipple area had scabbed and become irritated. I called Dr. S's office, and they asked me to come in. They saw me right away and told me I had a stitch infection. With it having been almost a year since my mastectomies, I thought all of my stitches had dissolved. I didn't realize I had a lot of internal stitches still inside me. Apparently one of the stitches became infected. The nurse cut the stitch, disinfected the area, and told me to put antibiotics on it twice a day for the next few days. The area healed just fine afterward. In my later research I discovered that after a mastectomy, one is sewn back in layers. Thus, if you have a mastectomy, you will have many internal stitches.

MY BRCA1 AND BRCA2 GENE MUTATION COUNSELING

August 27, 2007

A few weeks after meeting with the ob-gyn and discussing ovarian cancer and taking the BRCA1 and BRCA2 gene mutation test, I got a notice saying that if I wanted to meet with the gene counselor, I should call for an appointment within the next two weeks. I procrastinated and then scheduled my appointment. Mom, Gabby and Andrew went with me to meet genetics counselor Tammy on August 27, 2007, almost a year after my mastectomies. Tammy is very knowledgeable and informative. She asked us questions about our family tree on my mom and dad's sides. She asked who had what types of cancers and specifically wanted to know about melanomas, ovarian cancer and breast cancer. (Please see an in depth discussion of the BRCA1 and BRCA2 gene mutation in my section entitled Factors Which May Contribute to Whether You Will get Breast Cancer: Genetics-The BRCA1 and BRCA2 Gene Mutation" starting on page 138.)

Tammy told us the following:

- **10% of breast cancer is genetic and due to the BRCA1 or BRCA2 gene mutation.**
- **If you have the BRCA2 gene mutation you have a higher risk of melanoma.**
- **A female with the gene mutation may have up to an 87% risk of getting breast cancer during her lifetime.**

Based on my family tree, Tammy thought the possible gene mutation, would have been passed down on my father's side. I wondered why she didn't link it to my maternal grandmother who had breast cancer. Since grandma had not been diagnosed until in her 70's, and because none of her sisters or daughters had been diagnosed with breast cancer, she wasn't as strong a candidate. Alternatively, my father's side of the family is somewhat unknown because his mother's family died in the Holocaust. Thus, what cancers they had, or would have had, is unknown to us. My brother, Jonathan, has had three melanomas removed from his back and neck. Since this gene mutation creates a higher risk for melanomas, it is also a factor to be considered.

Tammy approved my having the gene test based on my breast cancer at an early age and my family history. My insurance plan paid for my testing. Myriad Genetic Laboratories in Utah performed the test, and you can contact the Myriad Reimbursement Assistance Program at 1(800)469-7423 to find out if your insurance will cover the test. Please see their website www.myriadtests.com for more information.

I next signed a consent form to have the "Hereditary Cancer Genetic Testing" done. Tammy also gave me a box from Myriad to take with me to the hospital. After they drew my blood, they would send it to Myriad. Tammy told me she would call a few weeks later to schedule a visit to discuss the results with her.

CHANGES AFTER MY DIAGNOSIS OF BREAST CANCER

I have panic attacks sometimes, even for the oddest reasons. By the way, I never had one before my breast cancer diagnosis. Every now and then I take half of a Xanax for anxiety. New aches and pains cause a lot more alarm than before. Thus, I have spent more time at the doctor's office than before my breast cancer. Due to my loss of confidence in my body's ability to stay healthy, I worry something serious could happen to me health-wise.

I tend to be compulsive about accomplishing things. When I start something, I'm determined to finish it. This perseverance is what helped me to get through my whole breast cancer ordeal. I also found projects to keep me busy like quilting which I began in January of 2007. Within one year I completed 10 quilts and pillows.

My cancer experience put things in perspective. We have limited time on earth. I wish I could say that after my diagnosis I lived each day as if it was my last day on earth, but I'd be lying. What I have realized is my best days are hanging out with my family and letting everyone do their own thing. I now appreciate what I have instead of what I don't have. I don't focus on the loss of my breasts because I still have my skin, I am so grateful not to have the cancerous tissue inside of my breasts. Instead, I have silicone shell implants filled with saline. As I've mentioned, they still feel like my boobs even though they are much harder to the touch than my old ones. When someone gets a limb replacement, do they suddenly feel less human? Some people have lost a lot more than I have, so I do not waste any time feeling sorry for myself. Of course, I'd rather not have gone through any of this yet I am grateful to have persevered through it as well as I have. I'll also accept letting go of my breasts before losing my life or suffering with full-blown cancer. I know that I made the right decision. When it is between my breasts or my life, I choose my life.

When asked by my friend, Laurel, what I had learned during my whole breast cancer experience, I replied, "Compassion."

Feeling the compassion of others toward me helped get me through my trying experience. I also learned to be more compassionate with others and to pay closer attention to others' needs. Relationships with people are what really matters. This is what helps us to get through the difficult times in life. Our belongings and things are nothing compared to the people in our lives.

MY SUPPORT SYSTEM:

In difficult times we learn who our friends really are. Some "friends" didn't call or make any effort to visit me. An acquaintance, Barbara, who I have known for many years organized friends to bring dinners over after my mastectomies. My best friend, Tanya, helped her coordinate the dinners. Seeing different people every night and knowing they cared eased my recovery. It also gave me a chance to talk about what I was going through. This helped my healing process both mentally and physically

Paul brought me flowers every Thursday, and vowed not to argue from my diagnosis in May until after my mastectomies in September.

I asked him if his kindness would continue after I'd healed. He replied, "No."

Well, at least he was there for me when I needed him to be. Although he hadn't agreed with my decision, he fully supported me throughout my having bilateral mastectomies. He never suggested I'd be less of a woman after a mastectomy. In fact, he likes my new breasts more than the old ones. Any man who would persuade a woman from getting a mastectomy, or who would feel she'd be less of a woman from having one, isn't worthy of being with you. As my grandpa used to say, "Don't let the door hit you in the ass on your way out."

My high school friends from Illinois, Debbie and Julie, sent me a beautiful bouquet of flowers after my mastectomies. My high school friend, Janet, mailed me a breast cancer blanket and a prayer from her church. My brother Jonathan sent me a beautiful plant arrangement and came out to visit me after my surgery. Paul's sisters Pauline and Janie, along with her partner Jan, brought a lovely plant arrangement. My brother Jeffrey visited me in the hospital after my surgery, and was available whenever I needed to talk. His ex-wife, Rita, also listened whenever I wanted to talk. My nieces Samantha and Teri cleaned my house; and Samantha took me for my stereotactic biopsy. My friend, Therese, purchased a membership for me to Netflix so I could have movies sent to the house during my down-time after the surgery. My neighbors, Charlotte and Dennis, Bill and Lisa, and Jackie brought me dinners and visited with me. My friends Jocelyn, Pam, Tanya and Carolyn and my business associate, Joy, also brought us meals and visited briefly. My neighbor, Teri, picked up my daughter from school, brought me plants and visited. Her daughter, Amanda, baked me brownies. My community of friends and family helped me to feel well-cared for and loved. Without them, I don't know how I would have made it through.

I remember calling my best friend, Tanya, on the day I received my breast cancer diagnosis. Within 20 minutes she showed up at my door with eight different types of Gatorade and a big bouquet of flowers. I had surgery scheduled two days later, and she knew I wasn't able to fast, so she brought me Gatorade to increase my energy. She wore her sunglasses in my house. I could tell she had been crying, and didn't want me to know. Tanya visited me in the hospital the night of my mastectomies and also drove me to the doctor for my nipple procedure. We met in law school in 1989 and have been close friends ever since. Everyone should have a friend as generous and supportive as Tanya.

I heard from my college room-mate, Jami, while in the fitting room with my daughter Gabby as she tried on her first training bra. I gave her the short version of my newly diagnosed breast cancer. So, as Gabby's boobs were developing, I would soon lose mine.

Another good friend from law school, Jocelyn, visited me in the hospital. She helped keep my mind off the surgeries. I preferred not to have too many visitors at the hospital and asked Paul and my Mom to limit them. Being hooked up to an IV and a catheter isn't exactly how I like to greet visitors.

Many family members stepped in to make things smoother for all of us. Paul's Aunt drove me to Dr. S's office for my injections of saline solution during my reconstruction, and I found it helpful to talk to her. She is a 20-year breast cancer survivor after doing radiation. Paul's sister, Pauline, drove me to Dr. S's office a few days after my mastectomies. Her cheerful presence lifted my spirits. She also spent the day with my mom and brother Jeffrey during my mastectomies/ reconstruction. She kept them calm and took their minds off of my surgery. Paul's other sister, Janie, came down from San Francisco to spent a day with me soon after my surgery which I so appreciated.

Friends continued to check on me. They seemed like my life-line. Julie, Debbie and Janet from high school in Illinois often called to chat and better understand my whole experience. Judy, from law school and Laurel, my room-mate from college, during an overseas program in Israel also stayed in close contact. Although far away, these ladies took the time to reach out to me with frequent calls and emails. This really helped me emotionally.

My doctor friend Brian, who I dated in my early 20's was very supportive. With a successful, internal medicine practice in Georgia, he still made time to email me, call me, answer all of my medical questions, and listen to my concerns.

My business associate, Mike, called every now and then to check on me. He is married to my "friend" who only called me once (returning my call a week after my mastectomies). Maybe she thought since I spoke regularly to her husband that I didn't need her support. Not quite the same.

My longtime friend, Tim, who can often be self-absorbed called several times to lend his support. We went for a long walk at the lake soon after my reconstructive surgery and had a very open talk about many topics including my breast cancer. I felt relieved to know he didn't think differently about me after my surgeries. Some other male business associates emailed me and called yet didn't seem to know what to say. My long time friend and mentor never responded when I emailed him about my breast cancer. I thought maybe he didn't get my email. I mentioned it a year later and he shared that he knew about it, but he thought it best not to bring it up. Not exactly the support you need.

As I think most women would agree, men think differently than woman. When we have a problem, many men think we want them to solve it. If they are unable to, they are at a loss of what to say or do. Women on the other hand, know sharing a problem is a way of venting and thinking out loud. We aren't necessarily seeking a solution. We just want to feel heard. Overall, I found women to be much more supportive than men. I guess it is in our genetic make-up.

We spent the day before my mastectomies, Labor Day, with our friends Carolyn, Joe, and their daughter, Lauren. She is Gabby's age and her best friend. Thankfully, it was a small gathering because I wasn't in the mood for socializing. Carolyn and I talked in the kitchen and both cried a little as we discussed the next, big day. She hugged me for a long while and wished me luck.

My friend Lynn, brought over chicken soup and challah bread after I came home from my second biopsy. She also visited me in the hospital after my mastectomies. She brought me a big basket with scented oils. I loved these surprises.

I am sad I had breast cancer, yet I discovered how many caring people I have in my life. My support system of friends and family is what got me through my entire breast cancer experience. The things people did for me, helped me emotionally. Many people want to help, let them. When someone is sick, they don't want to be ignored nor do they want pity. No one wants to be treated differently because they have the big "C", cancer. Respect all people as human beings with empathy. Know you can rely on the women in your life (and maybe some of the men in your life) to be there for you. If your loved one(s) have cancer, let them know you care. Call them, email them, bring them dinner, flowers, a plant, a card, or a little gift. No gesture is too small. All will be remembered. Don't miss out on an opportunity to get closer to someone. Let others be there for you, and be available for others when they need you.

So many people in my life know about my breast cancer and my mastectomies and thankfully no one treats me any different than they did before. You definitely don't want people looking at you like, poor so and so, she had breast cancer. Support is good but pity is not helpful.

I am so grateful for people like Dr. S who have dedicated their lives and careers to do the work they do. He is a caring artist with the ability to help a woman feel "whole", for lack of a better word. He's done reconstruction after skin saving mastectomies for about 18 years and is receiving national recognition for his results. He went to Berlin in the summer of 2007 to speak about the techniques and products he uses, along with, the results he has attained.

Dr. S's nurse, Barbara, and I became friends during the course of my procedures. She even came to my house and assisted me to rearrange and redecorate several rooms. What a kind and sweet lady.

July 21, 2007

To celebrate and thank all of the women who helped me get through my breast cancer experience, I hosted a tea for 23 women. Six more had been invited yet couldn't join us because they live in other states. Each one of these women and girls had done something special for me. I had the tea at my house and Paul's sister, Pauline, shopped and handled most of the preparation for this event. Gabby helped to set up our dining room and living room so we could seat all 23 of our guests. We used Grandma Syl's china that I ate on as a young girl. She'd had a mastectomy in her 70's so I found this most fitting. This way she could be with us in spirit. We placed out our fancy old teacups and saucers, and the tables had floral centerpieces that I made. I had sewn colorful sachets filled with lavender from my garden. Gabby and I had spent an hour or so picking the dried lavender and filling the sachets while mom hand-sewed the final little stitches. Each lady received one, along with, the silk orchid planter nearest their place setting.

When everyone had finished eating, I gave a thank you speech. Of course I had an outline so I wouldn't forget anything that I wanted to say. I shared that it had not been an easy year, yet due to all of their support and encouragement, I'd not only survived my experience – I'd thrived during it. I listed all of the things that everyone at the tea had done to support me during this time and that what had mattered to me the most had been all the love and caring everyone showed me. I acknowledged Pauline for all of her work on the tea and shared my deepest gratitude with Gabby and my Mom for changing my dressings for me, looking when I couldn't, and not being disgusted by what they saw.

I also shared how I relied on Gabby's strength. I told the story of us in the doctor's office when I felt uncomfortable about her seeing I had no nipples. I asked, "Would it bother you if I didn't have nipples?"

She replied, "No."

So I showed her my new breasts and she said, "It doesn't look bad mom. I thought it would look a lot worse."

I then told the ladies about how I became upset because Andrew's cried during his haircut and my smart little Gabby said, "You survived breast cancer mom, you can survive this." She has a way of putting things into perspective.

I thanked all of these dear women for caring so much for me in spite of their busy lives. Then I mentioned we had been eating on Grandma Syl's china. She had a place at the table with us in spirit. For anyone who may not have known, I told them about her breast cancer, mastectomy, and how she had chosen not to have reconstruction. When I told them about how she would take out her prosthesis for men or women to feel, they couldn't stop laughing.

Finally I told them about this book and urged them to call me if any of them knew someone with breast issues. Having already spoken to a few of them and to people they had referred to me, I'd been able to comfort and assist women with suspicious mammograms and also, breast cancer. I reiterated how much I had learned during this entire experience – all captured in my book to support other women experiencing this life wake-up call.

I thought I could be stoic and dry-eyed during my talk. With Tanya sitting next to me crying, my Mom crying, and a few of the other ladies tearing up; it wasn't possible. Letting myself have a good cry along with them gave me closure for all I had been through. It also felt so gratifying to stand in front of these compassionate women and shower them with appreciation. I'll never forget all they did to support me. They were my life-line. I only hope I can do the same for others.

FOLLOW-UP or lack of follow-up and LYMPHEDEMA

September 7, 2007

Today I had my follow-up visit with Dr. S. He said everything looked great. I pointed out some wrinkles/indented ridges primarily in my right breast with one ridge in the left breast. He indicated we could fix them by making incisions into my stomach, taking out some fat and then injecting it into my breasts. I would go under general anesthesia for this procedure. Since I couldn't handle any more anesthesia, I decided to leave the ridges alone.

Soon after this doctor's visit, I spoke to a friend who had DCIS and a mastectomy. She mentioned that she had the above procedure and, as a result, experienced a lot of pain in her stomach afterwards. She told me a lot of the fat that gets injected into the breasts dissolves or gets absorbed back into the body. (Why doesn't it absorb when it's in your tummy?)

September, 2007

I had originally been scheduled to see the general surgeon, Dr. X, who had performed my mastectomies, at the end of July of 2007. However, her office cancelled my appointment at the last minute because she got called into surgery. They added me to a wait list to see her but no one had called me. Dr. S's receptionist, Donna, was nice enough to check on Dr. X's schedule and found an opening for me on Monday, September 10, near my one year anniversary of my mastectomies. Since that time I had not had any follow-up other than my visits to Dr. S regarding the reconstruction. No one called me to discuss what I needed to do or not do, and Doctor X told me that I didn't need to see her again unless there was a problem. This didn't sit real well with me.

POINTS FROM DR. BARRY:

- Andrea was too hard on Dr X and her expectations of the Doctor.
- In the usual mastectomy scenario the general surgeon's role is to remove the breasts. Reconstruction and healing is for the plastic surgeon. And surveillance is for the oncologist.
- A problem with having DCIS, early stage breast cancer, may be follow-up. The surgeon may not think they need to do follow-up since they took the cancer out, and their job is technically done. The oncologist may feel they do not need follow-up since no chemotherapy was given.
- This can be confusing for the patient because she still feels she needs follow-up but doesn't know who to see.
- In the private world of medicine, the oncologist does follow-up and the primary care doctor and/or the ob/gyn doctor does the clinical exam (feel up).
- In an HMO, a busy surgeon may believe the patient is cured and will not want to see her again after removing the patient's breasts and only finding early stage breast cancer.

September 10, 2007

Today I met with Dr. X with my usual list of questions. My first and most urgent question involved my follow-up screening for a possible recurrence of breast cancer. She told me I did not need to have mammograms. A self-exam would suffice. She recommended

I get familiar with how my implants feel and then have my usual gynecological exam where the doctor examines my breasts. If I were to notice anything unusual, like a hard grain or lump, then I should come back to her; otherwise I don't need to see her again. (Dr. Barry doesn't think this is an unreasonable statement.) Dr. X did a fast breast exam since I insisted, and said everything felt fine.

Of course, everything about my breasts felt strange. I refer to them as MY breasts because that is how I regard them. It is still my skin, just different nipples, and the bad tissue has been taken out and replaced with implants. They do feel hard and bumpy; not soft and natural like a woman's breasts. They look great in clothes and fine naked, especially as my scars lighten.

I also expressed my concern to Dr. X about getting lymphedema, particularly since my fingers had been swollen since February of 2007. She said it is "not possible" to get lymphedema from the surgeries I had, and that was the whole point of performing the sentinel node biopsies.

POINTS FROM DR. BARRY:

- **Instead of saying it is "not possible" to get lymphedema after my mastectomies and removal of three lymph nodes, the better wording would have been "not likely."**

Dr. X also confirmed that I could return to all of my normal activities including getting blood pressure on my arm again. After the inaccurate high readings I had before, I felt quite relieved. I hoped Dr. X had given me the right information about lymphedema. I didn't want to get this. If we can't trust our doctors, who can we trust? Play it safe; each situation is different. Please check with your doctor(s) to see what you can and can't do.

In my research I have discovered even though the chances of getting lymphedema after a sentinel node biopsy are not as great as compared to a full dissection of axillary lymph nodes (the lymph nodes under your armpit), it is still possible. According to <u>Dr. Susan Love's Breast Book</u>, 4th edition, recent studies have shown if you have a sentinel node biopsy you have a 2-6% chance of obtaining lymphedema. This is considerably lower than the 17-34% chance of acquiring lymphedema if the full axillary dissection is done.

Something else I noticed for nearly a year after my surgeries, every time I washed, combed or ran my fingers through my hair, a lot more fell out than normal. I have always had a lot of hair so this troubled me. I asked Dr. S if hair loss from anesthesia is common. He told me some of his patients had mentioned hair loss. A breast cancer survivor, Joannie, also said she had lost a lot of hair after her surgeries. Then another person I spoke to, Bonnie, shared that she lost hair from the anesthesia during her knee surgeries. Perhaps it was the anesthesia that caused our hair loss or maybe just the stress of the situations that caused our hair loss, hard to tell.

Other than these concerns, after more than one year of having my mastectomies, I had fully recovered. Most of the feeling had returned in my breast areas and arms. I felt more pain yet nothing major. The pain increased as the feeling in my skin and breast area came back.

I believe I have done pretty much everything I can to minimize getting breast cancer again. Of course, I would be devastated if after all of my self-care, I get a recurrence of breast cancer. The reality I now understand is that until treatments become more conclusive for eliminating a recurrence for many types of breast cancer, mastectomy may still be the best option. For many types of breast cancer and for women with a higher risk, mastectomy may offer the least chance of recurrence. I believe opting for a mastectomy may provide the best chance of survival, though this has not yet been proven in scientific studies. If cancerous or potentially cancerous tissue is removed then it seems to me one's chance for a recurrence would decrease. Without a recurrence then how is it possible to die from breast cancer?

POINTS FROM DR. BARRY:

- **According to the December 2002 NCI Study, in stage I and stage II breast cancer, the survival rate was no different whether mastectomy or lumpectomy was performed. (Andrea says: You may want to read the study and draw your conclusions.)**
- **A lumpectomy may not be appropriate in very small breasted women, very large breasted women, or in women who have extensive DCIS.**
- **Andrea may feel that a mastectomy is the better choice of treatment for multifocal DCIS (early stage breast cancer in more than one area) but the Standard of Care for multifocal DCIS is still lumpectomy followed by radiation and possibly Tamoxifen or Aromatase inhibitors or a mastectomy.**

This could become a double-edged sword. If all women who are diagnosed with breast cancer choose to have mastectomies, how will treatment advances occur if ladies aren't willing to try new treatments or medications. Even after a mastectomy, other treatments may be necessary. Further, not all women will opt for a mastectomy, nor should they. Although a mastectomy may sound brutal and barbaric; it isn't, at least not in my experience.

December of 2008

I now felt something different along the scar tissue of my right breast. My finger appeared drawn to this area. I had my usual gynecological visit and the nurse practitioner shared how impressed she was with how my breasts looked. I had her feel the area which concerned me. She said it felt like normal scar tissue.

January 29, 2008

I met with my reconstructive surgeon, Dr. S, for a follow-up. After his exam, he shared that all felt fine. We discussed filling in some of the ridges in my skin. I told him my breasts looked great in clothes and good enough without clothing. I didn't want to undergo more surgery. He said I could get the ridges filled in at a later time and recommended I return in six months for my next visit. I told Dr. S about my concern with the scar tissue feeling more pronounced. After checking it, he thought it was only scar tissue. I told Dr. S I was nearly finished with my book and asked him if he would read it and give me his opinion. He said he would be honored to do so. Do all you can to find a compassionate person to attend to you in your time of need. Don't settle for less. You deserve only the best care.

February of 2008

It now seemed as if the scar tissue had become more pronounced, as if there was a small pebble near the scar tissue, of my right breast. So, on February 7th I called to make an appointment with Dr. X. With her busy schedule, I had to wait until March 10th for my appointment. My thoughts began racing again. I didn't look forward to my visit with Dr. X, yet I needed her expertise. If she had a bad attitude and acted like I am a nut for seeing her again I planned on asking her if she would prefer that I see another surgeon for future follow-up. I really don't think that seeing your surgeon every six months after a mastectomy is too often. I hoped that Dr. X would tell me it was nothing and just scar tissue. I wondered if I should rely on her expert touch or if I should request an ultrasound or some other screening device. (I didn't realize at this point that mammograms and ultrasounds would no longer be useful screening test for me since I no longer had tissue for them to look at.) I wanted to know that I didn't have a breast cancer recurrence. And if I did, I wanted to find it as soon as possible.

I wish I could tell you if you have your breasts removed you will live happily ever after and never think about breast cancer again. Perhaps you will learn to master your mind and tune out the thoughts about getting breast cancer again. It doesn't seem to work for me.

For the most part I don't dwell on the fact that I had breast cancer or may get it again. However, writing this book is a constant reminder for me. Almost everywhere I go I find something or someone who makes me think about breast cancer. There are many things in our life we can control but unfortunately, getting breast cancer is not one of them. What we can do is decrease our risks for getting breast cancer. (Please see the section of this book entitled "Factors that may contribute to whether you will get breast cancer," for pointers on what you can do to decrease your risk of getting breast cancer.)

March 10, 2008

I met with the general surgeon, Dr. X, who performed my mastectomies in September of 2006. According to Dr. X, follow-up is unnecessary. I just don't feel comfortable with this. If I had a recurrence, since I'd been diagnosed with high grade DCIS-non-invasive cancer, it could return as high grade quick spreading invasive cancer. As I've emphasized numerous times, by having the bilateral mastectomies I greatly reduced my risk of a recurrence, or new breast cancer, but after any type of breast cancer the thought of getting cancer again lurks somewhere in the mind.

Dr. X began our meeting with, "What can I do for you?"

I longed to hear, "How are you doing?", "Nice to see you,""You look great" or "Your breasts look good." I didn't even receive a friendly handshake. I took Xanax for four days before my appointment with her. She makes me feel like I am a hypochondriac making up symptoms. No, I am a woman who had her breasts cut off because that seemed like the most prudent treatment for early stage breast cancer that was in several locations in my breast. And after having my breasts cut off, I learned I had more early stage cancer which had not been detected before my breasts were removed. Why can't she respect my situation?

Dr. X mentioned she didn't feel anything besides scar, bone, rib cage and implant. I asked her if I should get an ultrasound to use as a baseline to compare to in the future. She told me an ultrasound wouldn't show anything bigger than 1 cm. My exit papers say, "return if symptoms worsen or fail to improve." If I don't have anything that is a problem, then what needs improving? Once again she didn't suggest any follow-up or monitoring. I left feeling as if I'd wasted her time, and definitely mine. Now I'd become determined to obtain a referral for a surgeon as equally skilled as Dr. X yet one capable of showing empathy and compassion.

Next my precious daughter, Gabby, joined me in my research. When I received the diagnosis s she was in 4th grade and 9. When in the 6th grade and 11 years old, she shared with me that she had a research project due for English class. She decided to research breast cancer and asked if it would be okay with me. Her teacher suggested she clear the topic with me. I thanked her for asking me and welcomed more support with my research. I shared some of my resources with her and she delved right in like a pro. She certainly knows a lot more about breast cancer than I did before my diagnosis.

Gabby used Dr. Susan Love's 620 page book entitled <u>Dr. Susan Love's Breast Book</u>, 4th edition, as one of her resources. She somehow opened it to an interesting section. It stated a possible, preventive measure of giving hormones to a teenage girl to induce a "hormonal pregnancy" for nine months with the theory that this will mature her breast tissue and thus, prevent breast cancer. (See page 192 of Dr. Love's book for more of an explanation.)

POINTS FROM DR. BARRY:

- **"Hormonal pregnancy" is an interesting concept but it has only been studied on rats so far and is controversial.**

The above theory suggests that the younger you are when you have your first child, the greater your protection against getting breast cancer. Of course, we don't want teenagers having a real pregnancy just to avoid breast cancer. If a fake pregnancy can be accomplished without too many risks and side effects, the potential to prevent or greatly reduce a girl's future risk of breast cancer is promising. (You may read Gabby's report at the end of this book.)

I feel sad that breast cancer is a part of Gabby's life. I pray there will be a cure before she gets older and may face it herself. I helped her research and edit her report, a fine piece of work for someone so young. Reading it upset me more than any of the other breast cancer resources I have studied. No mother wants breast cancer to be a part of her daughter's reality. I hope somehow that she doesn't fully understand she may be at a higher risk of getting breast cancer due to mine. We must do our part to encourage prevention and a cure, so my daughter and yours will never get breast cancer.

Unfortunately I read Dr. Love's book after my mastectomies rather than right after my diagnosis with DCIS. I visited her website and did other research after my diagnosis, yet found myself reaching a saturation point where I couldn't take in another thing on breast cancer. Therefore, I did most of my research after my mastectomies.

March 14, 2008

I came across some information in Dr. Susan Love's book which riled me up. In her discussion of "total mastectomy" which I believe I had, the removal of as much of the breast tissue as possible and some of the lymph nodes, she mentioned a woman can still get lymphedema. The chances of it are much smaller with a sentinel node biopsy, like I had, than when an axillary node dissection (removal of more lymph nodes) is done. According to page 456 of Dr. Love's book, recent studies show women who had sentinel node biopsies had lymphedema 2-6 percent of the time versus women who had full axillary node dissection getting lymphedema 17-34 percent of the time.

As I've discussed, in September of 2007, I told Dr. X about my swollen fingers and my concerns about getting lymphedema. She acted like I was crazy and said I COULDN'T get lymphedema. She didn't share there could be a slight chance of getting it and to exercise caution. Instead she flat out said I couldn't get it and for me to return to doing everything I had done before. Thus, I returned to getting blood draws, shots, and blood pressure in my arms. After reading Dr. Love's book I am taking the precautions I did before Dr. X assured me I couldn't get lymphedema. (See my discussion of lymphedema on page 190.)

Dr. Love mentions patients can have symptoms as minor as not being able to get their rings on. Well, I have had swollen fingers continuously since February of 2007, two months after my mastectomies and sentinel node biopsies.

March 25, 2008

I still hadn't taken the BRCA1 and BRCA2 gene test. I knew it would be wise to get the test, and I intended on having my ovaries removed if it showed I have either the BRCA1 or BRCA2 gene mutation. I just wasn't in the right place to absorb or act on the information. I did not want anymore surgery, namely having my ovaries removed if I had either gene mutation. I needed a chance to rest my body and my mind. If the gene mutation test turned out positive then I would schedule the removal of my ovaries right away. Ovarian cancer is almost always fatal, and there are usually no symptoms until it is far advanced. Unfortunately I've heard the CA 125 screening blood test is not a very good test for detecting ovarian cancer. Your tumor may not be producing a lot of CA125 so you may be falsely re-assured that you don't have ovarian cancer when you do have it.

During more research I wondered if my tissue had ever been tested to see if it was estrogen receptor positive or negative. I couldn't believe none of my doctors even brought this up. And if they had tested my tissue, why hadn't I been given the results? How would I know to request this? We rely on our doctors to order necessary tests. Do they request them? Do they even know about all of them?

POINTS FROM DR. BARRY:

- **Testing to see if breast tissue is estrogen receptor positive or negative is usually done only if invasive cancer is found.**

- **Historically such testing is not done for DCIS.**
- **Usually a sentinel node biopsy is not done for DCIS.**
- **Andrea had DCIS and a sentinel node biopsy was done.**

Through this research, I realized if I didn't know whether my tissue was estrogen receptor positive or negative, I couldn't make an informed treatment choice. If my tissue was estrogen receptor positive then radiation followed by Tamoxifen may have been an effective treatment for me. If I was estrogen receptor negative then it is very likely that Tamoxifen would have not given me much if any breast cancer prevention benefit. So, why take it and face the possible harsh side effects if I was going to get little or no benefit from taking it? If my lump/DCIS was estrogen receptor negative then it would not be as stimulated by estrogen as tissue that is estrogen receptor positive. Thus blocking estrogen from tissue that is not overly sensitive to estrogen doesn't really make sense.

POINTS FROM DR. BARRY:

- **Andrea's analysis about estrogen receptor positive and negative tissue makes sense intuitively but there has not been a study done about this, yet. Thus, there is no definitive scientific evidence to prove this.**
- **As of June 2008 testing the tissue to determine if it was estrogen receptor negative or positive was considered new and what to do with the results was still unclear.**

April 4, 2008

I found out that my tissue is estrogen receptor positive and that my progesterone is a weak positive because I asked the nurse practitioner to check what the computer showed about my tissue. Almost two years after my breast cancer diagnosis and long after my mastectomies, I learned that my tissue had been tested. I now knew the results. I still didn't know if it had been tested after my biopsies or my mastectomies. I suspect my biopsies were not analyzed for their response to hormones like I believe they should have been. The doctors didn't provide me with this information, so I could make an informed treatment decision. Again, we must be our own advocates. You must know the right questions to ask to get the right answers. (See my discussion of estrogen receptor positive tissue/tumors in "Treatment Choices.)

POINTS FROM DR. BARRY:

- **It does not matter if the tissue tested was tissue from the biopsy or the mastectomy. It was all basically the same tissue since the samples were taken pretty close in time. Thus all of the tissue would be either estrogen receptor positive or negative.**

I remember once asking my oncologist if I was estrogen receptor positive or negative, and he didn't seem to know. I happened to see this on a list of questions to ask the oncologist on a website I frequented. I had no idea what it meant until long after my mastectomies.

I recommend you have the lump/tissue taken during your biopsy analyzed to find out if it is estrogen receptor negative or positive, so you can make an informed treatment choice. Do not assume this is standard protocol. You don't want to select a treatment which isn't going to be effective for you. (I discuss this in more detail starting on page 216 in the section "How to make your treatment choices".)

As mentioned previously, Dr. X, the surgeon who performed my mastectomies, does not believe I need any follow-up to check for a breast cancer recurrence. Since I want a skilled professional to help me be watchful for a recurrence, as unlikely as it may be, I created my own follow-up plan with a nurse practitioner.

POINTS FROM DR. BARRY:

- **Perhaps Dr. X felt that she did not need to recheck Andrea and that an ob-gyn, primary care physician or oncologist could address her issues and provide follow-up.**
- **Sophisticated medical care requires a team with each person doing their job.**

I met with Nurse Practitioner, Alice, who had been highly recommended from my friend, Lynn. Alice works with the breast care center at my HMO, meets with women, and examines their breasts every day. She looked over my chart and told me she could not step on Surgeon X's toes by over-riding anything she did or did not do. I assured her I was not interested in doing that. I only wanted a plan in place for follow-up. She expressed concern over my being downgraded in my level of care from a surgeon to a nurse practitioner. I explained since I was not actually receiving any follow-up with the surgeon, this had become a moot point. Alice read through the notes from my last visit with Dr. X. She had written that I should return PRN, meaning as needed and with no follow-up date.

Alice immediately reached over and began a very thorough breast and chest examination. After reviewing the doctor's notes, she seemed to get my point. I'd been unaware that I should give myself a self-exam all over my breasts and chest area. I had only been concentrating on the area under my armpit by my scar. She emphasized how important it is to check the whole area. She did not find anything unusual, but if she did, it would feel hard like a knuckle. I asked for an ultrasound, and Alice said she couldn't order something unless Dr. X had requested it.

Alice assured me how unlikely it would be for me to get breast cancer again after my mastectomies and negative lymph nodes. She acknowledged me for being proactive about having a follow-up. I asked if she could refer me to a different surgeon who could provide follow-ups for me. She said she could not refer me to a different surgeon, yet I certainly deserved a second opinion. Thus, she would ask the Breast Care Coordinator, Judy, to call me with a referral. I shared how much I valued her opinions, and asked if I could see her again in six months. She agreed and even said I could come in before then if anything more urgent came up.

I asked Alice if she could tell from my records if my removed tissue was analyzed to see if it was estrogen receptor positive or negative. (I only knew to ask this because of the research that I had done for this book, after my mastectomies.) For the first time I learned that I was estrogen receptor positive and that my progesterone was a weak positive. I didn't ask her and she didn't tell me if this analysis was based on the tissue from my biopsies or from my mastectomies. I have a feeling that my biopsies were not analyzed for their response to hormones like I believe they should have been. If they were analyzed the results were never discussed with me as they should have been when I was trying to make an informed decision as to which treatment choice would work best for me. (See my discussion of estrogen receptor positive tissue/tumors in "Treatment Choices" starting on page 225.)

POINTS FROM DR. BARRY:

- **The above are controversial points not necessarily based in fact.**

Judy, the Breast Care Coordinator, called me later that day. I asked her for a referral for a surgeon as skilled as Dr. X but with a better bedside manner. I shared how pleased I'd been with Alice so I didn't need to see anyone right away. I planned on meeting with the new surgeon in the future. She gave me the name of a female surgeon who I'd schedule an appointment with in six months.

It still amazes me that a doctor would remove my breasts for early stage breast cancer and then not believe it necessary for any follow-up to make sure I don't have a recurrence. One would think a surgeon would understand that a woman who has had any type of breast cancer is always somewhat concerned about a recurrence. Even with a lower risk, I want a skilled medical professional to determine I am fine on a consistent basis. I do not want to leave my life up to chance. It is the only life I have.

I checked-out the NCCN practice guidelines in oncology and it doesn't recommend never having follow-ups again. For a pretty straight forward guideline, or standard of care regarding cancer in general, and specifically different types of breast cancer, please see the National Comprehensive Cancer Network, NCCN, website at www.nccn.org. Click on "NCCN Clinical Practice Guidelines in Oncology" and then go to your particular type of breast cancer. You can also go into "patients" and then "guidelines."

I still hadn't put breast cancer behind me. I continued doing research and ensuring I had follow-ups one and a half years after my mastectomies, nearly two years after my breast cancer diagnosis. If you have breast cancer, your life will never be the same either. Nonetheless do as much as you can to learn from the experience. It is a huge life lesson in standing up for yourself and being proactive with your self-care.

May 7, 2008

Almost two years after my diagnosis, I changed surgeons. As you know, I did not agree with Dr X's determination that I only need follow-ups for urgent matters. So, I met with Dr. K.

Dr. K said she would do follow-ups with me for five years based on my diagnosis and treatment. Since I had DCIS and my lymph nodes did not have cancer, she recommended I see her once a year for a physical breast examination. If I felt more comfortable with every six months, this would be fine. I chose to see her every six months.

She shared that even with a very low chance of recurrence, it is smart to follow-up. She performed a physical breast exam and assured me everything felt fine. The odd thing I'd been feeling was my rib poking out of scar tissue. She also said I do not have enough breast tissue to have an MRI, or an ultrasound, so my only screening is by physical examination.

I asked Dr. K about my concerns with lymphedema. She said it would be unlikely but anything is possible. She recommended I keep an eye on how the swelling in my fingers progresses. She also confirmed that my removed breast tissue was estrogen receptor positive. I asked her which tissue had been analyzed. She confirmed it to be the breast tissue from my re-excisional biopsy on May 12, 2006. (This information would have been helpful to know when I was making my breast cancer treatment decision.) I felt grateful for following my instincts. Although it took effort on my part, finding Dr. K had been so worthwhile. Make sure you take the time to connect with the right doctor for you.

November of 2008

I met with Dr. K again. She felt my chest and armpit area and determined all was well. This re-assurance by a doctor that I am doing well and do not have a lump boosts my mental well-being.

AN EMOTIONAL COMPONENT

Recently I told an acquaintance that I had nearly finished writing my breast cancer book. She had a lot of questions for me, and I had a lot of answers. After our discussion she asked if I had included an "emotional" component in the book. I think I forgot to breathe for a moment. Did she think my approach to breast cancer has been too analytical? Did she find it void of feeling?

I hope you will grasp in reading my story that my primary intention has been to treat this whole breast cancer subject as a research project. I tried to be as objective as possible in doing my research and in making my treatment decision.

If I thought too much about my choices, with the stress I experienced and the fear I felt, I am not sure I could have moved forward. Each of us gets through difficult situations in different ways.

Researching, seeking answers, and writing about what I have experienced, and learned has helped me get through this entire breast cancer process. I am still sad having a double mastectomy for early stage breast cancer seemed like the best treatment option available to me. I look forward to the day a cure for breast cancer is found. That will be the day I really allow myself to cry – for joy.

OTHER WOMEN I MET

Gabby invited her friend Amy to her birthday party in October of 2006. Her mom came in, and I met her for the first time. When she walked in, I'd been chatting with my friends about walking the Susan G. Komen Race for the Cure, a three day walk coming up in November, one month away. I asked Joannie if she'd like to join us. She said that since she had recently had a mastectomy, she would like to walk with us. I then noticed that she only had one breast. We stepped away from the group of ladies so we could talk privately.

Thankfully, I met Joannie after my mastectomies. She had also been diagnosed with DCIS. She had traveled a similar path as me by interviewing many doctors, asking many questions and doing a lot of research. She decided to have a mastectomy and reconstruction, yet opted for a single mastectomy instead of a bilateral mastectomy. She had her mastectomy about a month or so before mine yet continued to experience complications. She had swelling and drainage issues, so they removed her breast expander. I felt sad about what she was going through but almost didn't want to hear it. There can be risks and complications with any procedure. Over a year later, Joannie still had swelling and pain. I learned she had a permanent implant that the medical team may need to remove and also may need TRAMflap (tissue taken from the stomach to create the new breast) reconstruction.

My mom's friend, Edna, recently had a recurrence of breast cancer after having breast cancer 21 years prior. She had radiation after her first diagnosis. Now in her 80's she had to have a mastectomy. Thankfully, she managed through the procedure really well and is doing great.

I later met Cathy at a holiday party at a friend's house. I had heard about her from a friend. She was 45, going through a divorce, and had an 11-year-old daughter. It turns out she only lives a block away from me, this was the first time I ever met her. Wouldn't you know that at a party with 70 people, the two breast cancer survivor's are drawn to each other.

Cathy shared that she had been diagnosed with Stage 2 breast cancer about two years previously (or less). She had a lumpectomy, radiation, chemotherapy, and took Tamoxifen. Within a year she had a recurrence, and this time the cancer found its way into her bones and lymph nodes. She was undergoing chemotherapy again when I met her, and seemed to be handling it well.

She seemed like such a bright woman; however, she had not done any research on breast cancer. Basically her doctor told her what to do, and she did it. I don't know if she should have done anything differently, but my point is we must do our own research. This way we can look at ourselves in the mirror later and say, "Yes, I chose the right treatment for my situation."

It is important to listen to our doctors, yet we really must do our own independent research as well. You can do it! When you buy a car, a house, or any important purchase; don't you do some research? Aren't our lives worth it?

POINTS FROM DR. BARRY:

- **Things may not have gone differently for Cathy even with a mastectomy.**

In November of 2007, my niece's mother-in-law, Lucy, was diagnosed with Stage IV breast cancer. She was deemed "terminal". She felt a lump under her arm about a year before and had been too "busy" taking care of her older parents, children, and other people to get it checked. After her diagnosis, she started chemotherapy and lost all of her hair. After a year of treatment her MRI showed that her tumor had shrunk to half the size since before the chemotherapy. Everyone was hopeful. Unfortunately, as of June 2010 her breast cancer has spread to her jaw, brain, and many parts of her body. She is in hospice on a morphine drip and her days are numbered. She has been through so much. I feel terrible about what she has gone through. Take the time to take care of yourself! You need to come first, at least with your health. Without it you certainly cannot help other people.

Unfortunately, I have heard too many stories of women who delay their examinations or getting mammograms, even when they find something suspicious. DO NOT BE ONE OF THOSE WOMEN. It is much better to find breast cancer at an early stage than at a more advanced stage.

I have heard stories about doctors who don't do the testing because of either their incompetence, a woman's lack of persistence, or insurance issues. Be AGGRESSIVE. Take your life into your own hands. Demand testing, biopsies, and answers. Of course, before you know what to demand, you need knowledge.

Please talk to other women, read this book, do your internet research and definitely read <u>Dr. Susan Love's Breast Book</u>. Make sure you get the most recent edition, currently the 4th edition. Dr. Love's book is the bible on breasts and breast cancer. She is an expert. I am merely someone who experienced breast cancer and felt compelled to learn more about it. You don't need to spend the time or energy I have into studying breast cancer, but do enough research to find your answers and make the right decision for you.

Overall I'm in agreement with Dr. Love's viewpoints and the information she provides. She may think my decision to have a bilateral mastectomy for early stage, what some would call pre-cancer, multifocal DCIS was too aggressive. I made the right choice for me. You must make the choice which is right for you.

2. WHAT I LEARNED ABOUT BREAST CANCER

A. EARLY STAGE BREAST CANCER

- The breast is made up of two parts; the lobules which make milk and the ducts which are the branches that carry the milk to the nipple.
- If your breast cancer originates in the lobules, which are the ends of the milk ducts, then it is referred to as lobular carcinoma.
- It is thought that most breast cancer starts in the lining of the milk ducts. If your breast cancer originates in the milk duct itself then it is referred to as ductal carcinoma.
- Non-invasive or *in situ* breast cancer has not left the duct or lobule. It is contained in place (*in situ*- a Latin phrase) in the duct and/or in the lobule. So, non-invasive cancer can be ductal or lobular depending on where it originated. (I had non-invasive cancer in my ducts, DCIS.)

On the other hand, **invasive breast cancer is no longer early stage breast cancer**. It is breast cancer that has spread outside of the duct or the lobule where it originated and is now in other tissue or organs. However invasive cancer is still called ductal or lobular depending on where it originated.

a. DCIS (DUCTAL CARCINOMA IN SITU)

A theory is all breast cancer may start in the lining of the milk ducts. If your breast cancer originates in the milk duct itself, then it is referred to as ductal carcinoma. DCIS is basically clogged milk ducts.

In DCIS, there seems to be **a progression** from:

1. **a normal duct TO**
2. **intraductal hyperplasia which means too many cells in the duct TO**
3. **intraductal hyperplasia with atypia (also called atypical hyperplasia) meaning some cells look strange in the crowded duct TO**
4. **DCIS which is Ductal Carcinoma in Situ or intraductal carcinoma in situ meaning the cancer is in the ducts and in place (has not left the duct). These cells look abnormal, are crowding the duct, and multiplying.**

As one progresses along this spectrum, the risk of getting actual breast cancer increases. Numbers 2-4 above are considered pre-cancer because they are not YET invasive; however, it is believed they can become invasive cancer. Medical technology has not advanced enough to let us know if, or when, these early stage breast cancers will become invasive cancer.

Medical research estimates that 1/3 of DCIS BECOMES invasive cancer by DCIS cells eventually breaking out of the duct and spreading to nearby fatty tissue. I chose not to wait around to possibly become one of the 1/3 of women who had DCIS and later acquired invasive cancer. Thus, I took the drastic measure of having a bilateral mastectomy. Again, I made the best decision for me.

POINTS FROM DR. BARRY:

- **Andrea had multifocal (meaning found in multiple places) DCIS, nothing short of a mastectomy would get all of the DCIS out.**

What I still don't understand is if these stages are reversible. Can you be in # 3 above and go back to # 2 or 1?

Do cells look unusual at different times of the month because of hormones? Do they look out of the ordinary while pregnant or breastfeeding? I was told "no" that my breastfeeding had no bearing on the DCIS diagnosis I had been given. I'm still not sure I believe that. I also found out the stages are not reversible, yet I am not sure I believe that either.

POINTS FROM DR. BARRY:

- **We don't know if the stages are reversible. With DCIS you may or may not feel a lump.**
- **Usually DCIS is picked up as flecks of calcification in the ducts on mammogram.**
- **Symptoms such as a large mass, lumps in the armpit, skin ulcerations or arm pain are often a sign of advanced, Stage III or IV disease and not DCIS.**
- **DCIS is ductal carcinoma in situ. This is a bit confusing since carcinoma is technically cancer.**
- **Cancer is defined by a group of cells of one type which have gained the ability to grow and thrive amongst cells of a different type. Normally a cell of a particular type will stay with its own kind. (Think of cancer as integration of cell types as opposed to**

> segregation. A bad analogy since in society
> we tend to view segregation as bad and
> integration as good but you get my drift.)
>
> - **The most common cell type for breast cancer is ductal cell-the cells that normally line the ducts that carry milk from the glands to the nipple.**
> - **When the appearance of the ductal cell changes microscopically, yet the cell remains within the confines of the duct it is called DCIS.**
> - **When the changed cells begin to grow in other places in the breast outside the ducts, we call it invasive or infiltrating ductal cell carcinoma. The same can be said for Lobular Carcinoma in situ.**

DCIS is often symptom-free, and it generally does not show up on a mammogram. DCIS is a "pre-cancer" which is still in the CELL stage. It most likely has not yet formed into a lump. Keep in mind that mammograms and ultrasounds do not show CELLS.

DCIS is usually found by accident, like in my case it appeared next to a lump that kept returning. The lump had been benign, but it formed next to the DCIS. The thickening/lump I kept feeling may have been my clue that something wasn't right near it, i.e. DCIS had been developing in clogged ducts. It is similar to when you have an infection on your face and a whitehead or pimple forms. The pimple is an indication something is going on.

DCIS is more common than LCIS (Lobular Carcinoma in Situ). DCIS can grow into invasive breast cancer, but LCIS is not thought to become invasive cancer. Usually DCIS is not a lump but a soft thickening, like I had. I believe that this takes place because the ducts are no longer empty and soft as they should be. Instead they are filling up with cells. If DCIS does show on a mammogram, it may appear as micro-calcifications.

Most invasive breast cancer probably begins as DCIS cells. So, why does DCIS stay DCIS in some women and become invasive breast cancer in others? Studies are being done to resolve these questions. I believe the primary reason has to do with each woman's estrogen composition, and the absence or presence of the factors I discuss in the section entitled, "Factors which Contribute to Breast Cancer." Factors such as obesity, lack of exercise, a high fat diet, having the BRCA 1 or BRCA2 gene mutation, and alcohol consumption affect whether a woman will advance beyond the DCIS stage.

Perhaps the abnormal cells somehow break out of the milk ducts, make blood vessels to feed off of, and become invasive cancer. What causes this? Something may trigger or cause the cells to break-out based on what happens in your life over time coupled with your genetic or hormonal make-up. The cells may constantly attempt to leave to become invasive cancer, yet something keeps the DCIS from getting out of the ducts.

According to Dr. Sanford Barsky, a highly acclaimed breast pathologist and cancer researcher, myoepithelial cells sit near the ducts and produce enzymes which block the invasion of cancer cells. So, according to his theory, the abnormal cells are not leaving the duct because they CAN'T get out of the duct. (Thus, if they can get out, they will.) Why do some women's cancer cells get out of their milk ducts, and other women's cancer cells stay in their milk ducts? This prompted more inquiry.

If 1/3 of women who have DCIS later get invasive breast cancer, this means 2/3 of the women who get DCIS do not get invasive breast cancer. What makes these two groups of women different? The same factors may apply to both women either in a negative or positive way. Meaning perhaps the women who don't progress to invasive cancer are healthy, get enough sleep, eat right, don't drink too much alcohol, work out, don't take estrogen or hormone replacement therapy, and/or do not have the BRCA1 or BRCA2 gene mutation. Possibly the right combination of these factors prevent the cancer from becoming invasive.

Alternatively, women who do progress to invasive cancer may have allowed their resistance to go down for a period of time by not getting enough sleep, experiencing a lot of stress, eating a high-fat diet, drinking too much alcohol, taking hormones, and/or not exercising. They may also have had a recent pregnancy and breastfed, or have the BRCA1 or BRCA2 gene mutation. Potentially some, or all of these factors in certain women, may cause cells that weren't too active to get overly-stimulated and then break out of the duct, get into the fatty tissue surrounding the duct, thus, becoming invasive breast cancer.

The dormant abnormal cells may then eat through the proteins because they have gained the ability to do so; due to some combination of the above factors. Now they can go unchecked by the protective enzymes that had contained them. Possibly the protective enzymes' elimination over time allows the abnormal cells to break out of the ducts. This makes sense to me. What are your thoughts?

There are also grades of cancer. If a woman has low-grade DCIS and it becomes invasive breast cancer, it will most likely take longer to form than high-grade breast cancer. Thus, a woman may go a longer period of time before a recurrence of breast cancer when she starts out with low-grade DCIS as opposed to high-grade DCIS.

On the other hand, if high-grade DCIS becomes invasive breast cancer, it generally moves quickly and is more aggressive than low-grade invasive cancer. I had high-grade DCIS.

If you have been diagnosed with DCIS you need answers to the following questions: Is your DCIS multifocal, meaning in more than one area of the breast? Is it in different ducts, or the same duct, but a different region of the breast?

The breast is made up of two parts - the lobules which make milk and the ducts which are the branches that carry the milk to the nipple. There are five to nine ductal systems in each breast, and they do not connect to each other. One ductal system can be in several areas or quadrants of the breast. Thus, DCIS can appear to be in more than one ductal system when actually it is the same ductal system in more than one quadrant of the breast. Of course, I found this out after my mastectomies.

It may seem as if you have multifocal DCIS because the DCIS is found in more than one area, yet it is possible the DCIS is only in **one ductal system** within different regions of the breast. Not DCIS in multiple ductal systems. So, find out from your doctor and/or pathologist if your multifocal DCIS is believed to be in two DIFFERENT ducts or two different sections of the same duct. This is important in knowing how widespread your DCIS is and which treatment choice is most appropriate for you. If you have DCIS in many ducts, thus spread through-out the breast, you may want to consider a mastectomy, as I did.

POINTS FROM DR. BARRY:

- **Whether your multifocal DCIS is in two DIFFERENT ducts or possibly two different sections of the same duct can not be determined prior to mastectomy and it may not be determined at the time of a mastectomy either.**

IF YOU HAVE BEEN DIAGNOSED WITH *MULTIFOCAL DCIS (DUCTAL CARCINOMA IN SITU* IN MORE THAN ONE PLACE) THEN READ THE ABOVE PARAGRAPHS AND THE NEXT FEW PARAGPRAPHS CAREFULLY, SEVERAL TIMES, AND DISCUSS THEM WITH YOUR DOCTOR, BEFORE YOU MAKE YOUR TREATMENT CHOICE.

It almost seems easier to have a lump, even a big cancerous one, than several areas of DCIS in different ductal systems. What I mean is, they may be able to remove the whole cancerous lump with a clean margin around it, and then you may not need any more treatment. Yet, with DCIS, **abnormal cells**, these can be found in other areas of the same ductal system or in other ducts. Thus, they can spread around your ductal system. If you are diagnosed with *multifocal DCIS,* know your scenario before you make your treatment choice.

POINTS FROM DR. BARRY:

- **The above are odd statements since the prognosis of someone with DCIS is better than for someone with a big cancerous lump.**

In the mammogram I had after my *multifocal* (more than one area) *DCIS* diagnosis, small calcifications were scattered around both of my breasts. It is possible some were DCIS. After this mammogram I had a stereotactic biopsy to remove the most suspicious calcifications in each breast. The tissue samples came back showing no signs of cancer. Yet the pathology report after my mastectomies indicated I had a 2.5 centimeter area (about an inch) of DCIS that my mammogram or ultrasound did not detect. It also did not show up in both self-exams and examinations by my doctor, and had not been removed during my multiple biopsies. Had I not had the mastectomy, it may have gone un-detected for a long time. Scary. Remember CELLS cannot be seen in a mammogram or ultrasound, and abnormal cells cannot be felt.

If I hadn't chosen the mastectomies, and the DCIS had been found later, we probably would have determined it a recurrence. If you have DCIS, and then acquire it again, it may not be a recurrence. It could be left behind DCIS which has gone un-detected. Even though you may have had a clean margin (enough area around the DCIS deemed DCIS or cancer-free) around the original DCIS, it is possible more DCIS lurked in an area far enough away from the original biopsied region to go unnoticed.

As I've emphasized, I believe a mastectomy gives the lowest rate of recurrence when one is diagnosed with multifocal DCIS. Your surgeon can take out as much of your tissue and cells as possible. If all of the DCIS is removed, then it does not have the opportunity to become invasive breast cancer.

According to <u>Dr. Susan Love's Breast Book</u>, 4th edition, with DCIS the chance of a breast cancer recurrence after mastectomy is 1-2% and with breast conservation or wide excision there is a 5-10% chance of a recurrence.

Dr. Love states dying of breast cancer has a risk of 1-2% for either of these procedures. I am not sure why all of the procedures would give the same risk of dying. I remember my surgeon also telling me the studies did not indicate any higher rate of survival after a mastectomy, as compared to having the area of DCIS removed, coupled with getting radiation and taking Tamoxifen.

Doesn't it seem that a lower rate of getting a recurrence would also mean a reduced risk of dying from breast cancer? If we don't get breast cancer again, then how do we die from it?

b. LCIS (Lobular Carcinoma in Situ)

- **If your breast cancer originates in the lobules, the ends of the milk ducts, then it is referred to as lobular carcinoma.**
- **LCIS, Lobular Carcinoma in Situ, is a pre-cancer. The lobules normally don't have cells in them, but, in LCIS, the lobules are filling up with small, round cells.**
- **It is thought that most lobular breast cancers are sensitive to hormones. Your tissues' sensitivity to hormones is important to determine which treatment choice will work best for you.**

Like DCIS, LCIS, also follows a progression. The progression can go from:

- **normal lobules. TO**
- **lobular hyperplasia, a few normal cells are in the lobule. TO**

- **atypical lobular hyperplasia (ALH), the lobule becomes full of cells, and the cells begin to look abnormal. TO**
- **LCIS , Lobular Carcinoma in Situ, the lobule is filling up with abnormal or atypical cells.**

These abnormal cells in the lobules will most likely not become invasive cancer; however, they are an indication that something unusual is occurring in the breast.

If you are diagnosed with LCIS, you have several treatment options including: prophylactic double mastectomies; watching carefully which may include mammograms and self-examination; or taking Tamoxifen for five years if you are premenopausal, and your LCIS is estrogen receptor positive. If you are diagnosed with LCIS and are postmenopausal and estrogen-receptor-positive, then you may want to consider taking an Aromatase Inhibitor or Tamoxifen followed by an Aromatase Inhibitor. Weigh out all of the risks and benefits for each option very carefully with your doctor. Also take some time to decide on your own what is right for you. (Please see my sections entitled "Treatment Choices" and "How to Make Your Treatment Decision" for a more thorough discussion. See pages 177 and 216.)

To clarify, I had DCIS, so my research primarily focused on DCIS. Please do additional research if you get a diagnosis of LCIS.

B. FACTORS WHICH MAY CONTRIBUTE TO WHETHER YOU WILL GET BREAST CANCER

- **Age**
- **Breast density**
- **Pregnancy**
- **Breastfeeding**
- **Fertility drugs**
- **Hormones, especially estrogen**
- **Number of lifetime menstruation cycles**

- **Menopause**
- **HRT-Hormone Replacement Therapy for menopausal symptoms**
- **Weight**
- **Diet**
- **Exercise**
- **Alcohol consumption**
- **Environmental factors**
- **Genetics-the BRCA1 and BRCA2 gene mutation**

Many factors contribute to whether a woman will get breast cancer. Not one thing causes breast cancer, if so scientists would have easily found a cure by now. I believe it is the interaction of many factors, and your body's response to these factors, which affects whether or not you will acquire breast cancer. You will not cause your breast cancer but there are certainly things you can do to lower your risks of getting breast cancer. Unfortunately, even if you take the best care of yourself and do everything possible to lower your risks, you can still get breast cancer.

Many of the factors are known. Everyone should decrease as many known, negative factors as possible and enhance their immune systems. I don't think the exact same factors will have the same response in all women. As women, none of us are exactly like, and we all respond differently. For example, you may get hives when you eat tomatoes. This doesn't mean all women do, but somehow your body has an allergic reaction to tomatoes. It may be similar with the factors contributing to breast cancer. Some women will react to the factors and get breast cancer, and others will not.

It seems women may be more susceptible to getting breast cancer when they are breastfeeding, pregnant, a recent mom with a new baby, tired, stressed, overweight, eating a high fat diet, or drinking a lot of alcohol. (Factors can apply to most of us in different combinations.) It could be like catching a cold or the flu. You may come into contact with the germs which will give you a cold or the flu. Yet you don't contract it unless your resistance is down (i.e. you are stressed, not getting enough sleep, not exercising, or eating right). This may suggest that building up our immunity as much as possible can help us to avoid getting breast cancer and other illnesses. We need to treat our bodies like well-oiled, maintained machines. Without them, where can we live?

AGE

- **The older you are the higher your risk for breast cancer.**
- **About 80% of breast cancer is found in women who are over 50 years old.**
- **Women under 40 years old usually have dense breasts and a mammogram may not show anything, even though the woman or her doctor may feel something suspicious.**

Sometimes women under 40 are told nothing is wrong or to wait and watch. If women under 40 get breast cancer, it may be aggressive and even more so if they were pregnant within the last four years.

The risk for breast cancer is highest right after pregnancy and decreases over the next four years. Why is this? Apparently your milk ducts and hormones are greatly affected by pregnancy.

BREAST DENSITY

- **It seems there is a correlation between breast density and breast cancer.**
- **If you decrease the breast's density by using drugs like Tamoxifen, you may decrease your risk for breast cancer.**
- **Most young women have denser breasts that get fattier as they age, thus less dense.**
- **If you have dense breasts after menopause then this may increase your risk for breast cancer.**

I'd been told often I had dense breasts. I never thought about it because when we are young, our breasts are supposed to be this way. My dense breasts could have been an indication of an increased risk for breast cancer.

PREGNANCY

- **During pregnancy a woman's level of progesterone and estrogen changes along with other hormones to create milk.**
- **Besides being attractive, the female breasts' main purpose is to produce milk for a child.**

I heard Dr. Susan Love, the author of <u>Dr. Susan Love's Breast Book,</u> which is the bible on breast cancer, speak on the TV show, <u>The View</u> on October 17, 2007. (I don't usually watch TV during the day but my brother, Jeffrey, called to suggest the show.)

According to Dr. Love:

- **The female breast is not fully mature until it has gone through a nine month pregnancy cycle.**
- **Women who have a child before age 35 have a lower risk of getting breast cancer than women who have never been pregnant.**
- **Women who have their first child after 35 have a higher risk of getting breast cancer than women who have never been pregnant.**
- **The earlier you are pregnant the better it is for decreasing your risk of breast cancer.**
- **Ladies of higher socio-economic classes who are busy going to school and establishing their careers have an increased risk of breast cancer because they have children later in life.**

So, if you want to improve your odds for staying free from breast cancer then have your first child before the age of 35 or don't get pregnant after 35. I wondered if this meant I was a wash since I had one child before 35 and the other after 35.

Even if you have your kids early, stay alert for any suspicious lumps or something that just doesn't feel right. Take note of this. Again, women diagnosed with breast cancer during pregnancy, or within four years of childbirth, can get very aggressive cancer, probably because a normal, viable pregnancy involves a woman's estrogen and other hormone levels going up substantially. Thus, if you are moving toward breast cancer, this extra boost of estrogen may push you into full-blown, invasive breast cancer.

As I've discussed earlier, a little chart in the literature given to me about the HALO NAF test (See my chapter on Screening Tests for more discussion on the HALO NAF test.) sent me into a tizzy. It states the "Diagnosis of breast cancer within two years of childbirth has close to a 50% mortality rate." (Keep reading for clarification.) This came from, "The Relation of Reproductive Factors to Mortality from Breast Cancer" and is found in <u>Cancer Epidemiology Biomarkers and Prevention</u>, Volume 11, pages 235-241 from March of 2002. The article was written by Janet R. Daling Kathleen E. Malone, David R. Doody, Benjamin O. Anderson and Peggy L. Porter.

I looked this article up on the internet (see <u>http://cebp.aacrjournals. org/cgi/content/abstract/11/3/235</u>) and read the study. It mentions that 48.2% of women with **INVASIVE** breast cancer within two years of having a baby died of breast cancer. 1174 women were studied. I am not sure this is a large enough group of women to draw such firm conclusions. You will need to read this for yourself, and also, see some of the other related studies to draw your own conclusions. Thoroughly discuss this with your doctor if you fall into the category of having a child within the last two years, with a diagnosis of breast cancer, especially **invasive** breast cancer during or after childbirth.

Learning that 48.2% of women who get diagnosed with breast cancer within two years of having a child will die of breast cancer, upset me. I called my doctor friend, Brian, about it. He pointed out they said **"INVASIVE"** breast cancer, and my cancer was not invasive. I felt a little better but was still upset.

You MUST take this warning and the above statistic seriously, especially if you are pregnant or have recently been pregnant. If your doctor thinks your breast problem is just an infection or something minor, make sure he or she is absolutely right. We're talking about your life if they are wrong.

I recommend another article, "Effect of reproductive factors on stage, grade and hormone receptor status in early-onset breast cancer," by Joan A. Largent, Argyrios Ziogas and Hoda Anton- Culver, written in 2005. It can be found online at: http://breast-cancer-research.com/content/7/4/R541. It states "women younger than 35 years (old) who are diagnosed with breast cancer tend to have more advanced stage tumors and poorer prognosis than do older women. Pregnancy is associated with elevated exposure to estrogen, which may influence the progression of breast cancer in young women." Only 298 women participated in this study. This sampling could be too small to draw such firm conclusions. Nonetheless, if you are younger than 35, or recently pregnant when you get diagnosed with breast cancer, then you may want to read this article.

The risk for breast cancer is highest soon after your pregnancy and decreases over time. Studies indicate **death** from breast cancer is higher in women who have been pregnant within four years of their breast cancer diagnosis. You certainly don't want to have a new child and then die. Take preventive measures, schedule your examinations, and do your self-exams. If you are diagnosed with breast cancer, then don't be afraid of the treatment. It can save your life.

According to page 152 of the 4th edition of Dr. Susan Love's Breast Book, a woman has a greater risk for breast cancer during pregnancy and for ten years following it. Isn't that comforting news? I thought pregnancy decreased the risk of getting breast cancer. Since during pregnancy a woman's body boosts the production of estrogen and other hormones, this increases the risks for breast cancer. Pregnancy also causes greater cell division.

Although it seems as if the above statements regarding risks for four or ten years contradict one other; I don't think this is the case. My understanding is a woman's risk for breast cancer can be higher for ten years following her pregnancy, and the risk of death from breast cancer is greater if she has been pregnant within the last four years.

Estrogen is a hormone produced by the ovaries, adrenal glands, placenta, and fat. In terms of the placenta producing estrogen, when you are pregnant you have one growing inside of you. Since it creates estrogen this may explain why you have an increased risk for breast cancer up to ten years after your pregnancy.

If your breast tissue is estrogen-receptor-positive making it sensitive to estrogen, or you have the BRCA1 or BRCA2 gene mutation, (see the discussion of these in their section) you are already at a higher risk for breast cancer. Thus, the extra boost of hormones and hormonal fluctuations during your pregnancy may contribute to your getting breast cancer during or after your pregnancy.

If you feel or notice anything suspicious with your breasts during pregnancy, or for four to ten years after childbirth, get it checked right away. Do not put this off; it could mean your life. Do not allow a doctor to dismiss you because you are young or just had a baby. Make sure you err on the side of caution and seriously consider getting a biopsy for anything which seems out of the ordinary. Please talk to your doctor and aggressively pursue any abnormality to make sure that it is either not cancer or if it is cancer that you figure out the treatment choice that gives you the best chance of survival. You want to be alive to take care of your new baby.

If you are diagnosed with breast cancer during pregnancy, then you must ask your doctor to explain all possible treatments you can receive while pregnant, along with, how they will affect you and your fetus. Different choices are available depending on which trimester you are in.

In summary:

- **The earlier you have your children, the more breast cancer protection you will have.**

- Your risk of getting breast cancer is higher after pregnancy and decreases over time.
- You must make sure that any breast abnormality is not breast cancer.
- If you do get breast cancer, particularly invasive cancer within a few years of being pregnant, then you must aggressively seek treatment since the risk of death is very high for at least the first two years. It isn't easy for me to be in your face with this information, but you must be aware of this and do all you can to stay alive.

POINTS FROM DR. BARRY:

- Late in life pregnancy is almost like never getting pregnant in terms of increasing the risk of getting breast cancer.
- Nulliparity, never getting pregnant, may increase the risk of getting breast cancer.
- Early pregnancy correlates with a lower risk of developing breast cancer.

BREASTFEEDING

- Breastfeeding helps decrease the risk of getting breast cancer, so it seems the longer you breastfeed - the more protection you receive.
- When you breastfeed you may not get your period. Am I the only one who didn't know this?

I breastfed my first child for about five weeks, not much breast cancer protection. I nursed my second child for 18 months, but by then I may have been well on my way toward DCIS given I had atypical cells about two years before my second pregnancy, This was about four years before my DCIS had been diagnosed.

Either breastfeeding did not protect me, or maybe my breast cancer would have been worse if I hadn't breastfed for 18 months. Not having a period for 18 months, while breastfeeding, with fewer ovulation cycles thus, fewer hormonal cycles, should have decreased my risk for breast cancer.

FERTILITY DRUGS

- **Talk to your doctor about your personal increased risk for breast cancer if you take fertility drugs to get pregnant.**
- **Make an informed decision based on the risks and benefits of taking fertility hormones.**

HORMONES

- **Controlling estrogen appears to be central to preventing and/or managing breast cancer.**
- **Women's hormone levels change as they get older - monthly and during pregnancy.**

ESTROGEN:

According to the National Cancer Institute website http://www.cancer.gov/cancertopics/aromatase-inhibitors, "Many breast tumors are 'estrogen sensitive', meaning the hormone estrogen helps them to grow. Aromatase Inhibitors can help block the growth of these tumors by **lowering** the amount of estrogen in the body. Estrogen is produced by the ovaries and other tissues of the body, using a substance (an enzyme per Dr. Barry) called aromatase." (See my discussion on, "Medications for Postmenopausal Women-Aromatase Inhibitors.)

If the ovaries produce estrogen then it would seem removing one's ovaries would decrease the risk for breast cancer. (See my discussion of this under the Gene Testing section in this book.) Did you realize your ovaries are a main source of your estrogen production? I didn't until writing this book.

Since women and men have different hormonal compositions, women are more likely to acquire breast cancer than men. I believe it is our hormonal composition which has us at more risk for breast cancer. Perhaps it is the mere fact we are women, often under more duress, that causes us to get breast cancer.

POINTS FROM DR. BARRY:

- **Men without a BRCA1 or BRCA2 gene mutation, have about a 1% chance of getting breast cancer.**

In my opinion, your own personal level of estrogen, and in particular your estrogen level fluctuations over time, is a major factor, if not "the major" factor, in determining whether you will get breast cancer, and if you do, the treatment which will be right for you. (See my discussion of estrogen-receptor-positive tumors in the section entitled "Treatment Choices.")

THINGS WHICH MAY PRODUCE TOO MUCH ESTROGEN:

- **Estrogen replacement therapy**
- **Diet – eating too much red meat or chicken especially if the animal consumed hormones**
- **Alcohol**
- **Not enough exercise**
- **Not enough fiber in your diet**
- **Too much fat in your diet**
- **Being overweight (fat stores estrogen)**
- **Being someone who produces a lot of estrogen**

PMS AND HORMONAL FLUCTUATIONS

Controlling our hormonal imbalances as much as possible is helpful in relieving PMS as well as decreasing our risk of getting breast cancer. PMS symptoms probably arise out of an imbalance of too much estrogen and not enough progesterone. This is more likely the situation in the second half of the menstrual cycle, 14 days before a woman's period referred to as the luteal phase.

Here are some ways to relieve PMS and hormone fluctuations:

- **Decrease sugar, salt, and caffeine intake especially two weeks before your period. (I sure do crave chocolate the week before my period. You?)**
- **Keep your blood sugar balanced by eating four to six small, healthy meals every day. Have breakfast, lunch and dinner with one to three small snacks in between. This also helps you avoid binging and overeating.**
- **Eat a high fiber, low-fat diet with a lot of fruit, vegetables, whole grains, and fish.**
- **Decrease junk food, fatty and fried foods, and don't have too much dairy.**
- **Exercise is very important. (See the book <u>The Abs Diet for Women</u> by David Zinczenko for helpful exercise and eating suggestions.)**
- **Exercise will increase your endorphins, the "feel good" chemicals which go to the brain, especially after or during aerobic exercises when your heart rate increases.**
- **Exercise may decrease your PMS symptoms and estrogen levels, stabilize your blood sugar, and reduce your stress level.**
- **Consider taking:**

- **Calcium.**
- **Magnesium.**
- **Vitamin B6.**
- **Vitamin E.**
- **the herb, Black Cohosh, reported to decrease PMS symptoms and balance your hormones.**
- **the herb, Dong quai, noted to help balance your hormones and decrease breast tenderness and cramping.**
- **and the herb, Chasteberry, thought to help decrease the symptoms of PMS, and mood swings, as well as promoting the correct ratio of estrogen to progesterone.**

Check with your doctor before taking any of these vitamins or herbs!

HOW DOES ESTROGEN COME INTO PLAY?

I believe the key to understanding breast cancer lies in studies related to estrogen, other hormones, and how they interact and fluctuate throughout different cycles of a woman's life. Womens life cycles include development, puberty, menstruation, pregnancies, breastfeeding, and menopause. The earlier you menstruate and the later you begin menopause increases your risk for getting breast cancer. Thus, there is a connection between the number of menstrual cycles you have over your lifetime, and your risk of getting breast cancer. Essentially, the more periods you have - the more your risk increases. This relates to why removing your ovaries decreases your risk of getting breast cancer. Without your ovaries, you do not go through a menstrual cycle.

After menopause a woman's natural estrogen levels are most likely lower than at other times of her life. SO, WHY DO MORE POSTMENOPAUSAL WOMEN GET BREAST CANCER THAN PREMENOPAUSAL WOMAN?

Your likelihood of getting breast cancer over your lifetime increases as you move along the age spectrum. Thus, older women are more likely to get breast cancer than younger women since they have experienced more hormonal fluctuations during the course of their lifetime.

I also found information indicating many women have an increased level of estrogen and testosterone after menopause. (This contradicts what I just told you a few sentences ago.) After menopause a woman's ovaries do not produce much estrogen; however, other parts of her body can begin to increase their estrogen production. This may be to compensate for the decreased production of estrogen by the ovaries.

In postmenopausal women an enzyme called aromatase takes other hormones and turns them into estrogen. Thus, the recent development of drugs called Aromatase Inhibitors (they help women halt their creation of estrogen from other hormones.) (See my discussion of Aromatase Inhibitors in the section entitled "Treatment Choices." See page 200.) This increase in hormones results in postmenopausal women having a greater risk for breast cancer. Stopping the production of certain hormones (particularly estrogen) should help decrease the risk of getting breast cancer for these women.

One would think there would be a way to measure a woman's level of estrogen and other hormones at different stages of her life, i.e. soon after she gets her period for the first time, during pregnancy, during breast-feeding, pre-menopause, at menopause and post-menopause. Perhaps hormone testing at a set interval of every year or two would make the most sense. Thus, if hormones are a direct link to breast cancer, checking an individual's particular hormone levels could be a regular screening test like a mammogram or a Pap smear.

It seems like we should be able to examine hormonal levels the same way we measure sugar levels for a diabetic. Maybe researchers could tell us at X estrogen levels you are increasing your rate of breast cancer by "z." Thus, you need to reduce your estrogen by "x-3" or whatever the "normal" level of estrogen for you is determined to be.

Perhaps a self-test will be developed, like diabetics have, to monitor the hormone levels for all women, especially those at a higher risk for breast cancer. Reaching the ideal balance of hormones could mean other hormones need to be increased, or a woman needs to change her diet, exercise more, lose weight, or do something else to change her hormonal balance, **without** taking hormone replacement therapy.

I believe controlling a woman's hormone levels is critical to controlling breast cancer. I do not encourage artificial hormones to balance her out. I envision the hormonal balance being reached through natural ways.

There are many articles and studies about hormones, yet many are confusing and in scientific language. You can search the internet and find plenty to read.

OVARIES

- **If you have ovaries you experience hormonal cycles, even without a period.**
- **Not having your period anymore means you will have inconsistent hormone levels (as you will likely agree with if you are in this age bracket).**

I have confirmed with my research that removing our ovaries decreases the risk for breast cancer. The ovaries are a major if not "the major" producer of a woman's hormones. If you have your ovaries removed, and do not take hormone replacement therapy, you will decrease your production of hormones. Studies indicate this also decreases your risk for breast cancer. (See my discussion of having an oopherectomy (ovaries removed) in the BRCA1 and BRCA2 gene section of this book.)

There is no easy solution. By removing both ovaries you lose the production of some hormones, so your menopausal symptoms could be worse. On a positive note, you should decrease your risk for breast cancer by removing them.

OSTEOPOROSIS AND ESTROGEN

- **Dr. Susan Love points out that in postmenopausal women there seems to be an inverse relationship with breast cancer and osteoporosis.**

According to the 4th edition of <u>Dr. Susan Love's Breast Book</u>, in postmenopausal women, women with osteoporosis have 60% less breast cancer than women who do not have osteoporosis. She attributes this to a woman's natural level of estrogen. If you have lower levels of estrogen in your body, you may increase your risk for osteoporosis yet decrease your risk for breast cancer.

It seems there is a need for a drug which decreases a woman's estrogen level in order to give her breast cancer protection. Then she can be treated for osteoporosis with calcium or other supplements. This could likely help women who are at high risk for breast cancer. I haven't had osteoporosis so I don't have first-hand information on it, yet at least it isn't deadly as breast cancer can be.

NUMBER OF LIFETIME MENSTRUAL CYCLES

- **The more ovulation cycles (periods) a woman has during her lifetime, the higher her risk of breast cancer.**

The length of time I am referring to is between the age of menstruation and when you stop getting your period. The more ovulation cycles a woman has, the more cycles of hormonal fluctuations she will have. (It is normal to have fluctuations at different times of the month.) I am sure most women will agree they feel different at various times of the month. Hormonal changes are often the cause

Research suggests if you menstruate for more than 40 years, your risk of breast cancer goes up substantially compared to someone with fewer ovulation cycles and less hormonal fluctuations. Hormonal fluctuations appears critical, leading to why more postmenopausal women have breast cancer than premenopausal women. I haven't experienced menopause yet, though I've heard our hormones can really fluctuate and often become unbalanced.

PERIMENOPAUSE

- **Perimenopause includes the two to eight years before menopause begins and the first year of menopause.**
- **During this time frame the production of the female hormones estrogen and progestin decrease. Symptoms can include: hot flashes; urinary problems; mood changes (I can relate); sleeplessness; and shorter and lighter, or lighter and longer periods.**
- **Symptoms often start in the mid-40's yet can be earlier or later.**
- **Symptoms often stop when your menstrual period ends, yet then new symptoms may arise.**

MENOPAUSE

Women who menstruate for more than 40 years seem to be at a higher risk for breast cancer. For example, a woman who began her period early, at 10-12 years old, and goes into a late menopause (in her 50's) can be at a higher risk than someone with a shorter time frame of periods. It seems the longer you have cycles of varying hormones, the greater your risk for breast cancer.

Women reach menopause in three ways:

1. **Natural menopause.**
   - **It is your body's time to go into menopause.**
   - **If you still have your ovaries after menopause then they will continue to produce hormones yet at a lower level than before menopause.**

- **The later your natural menopause, the more your risk for breast cancer increases due to the greater length of time your body undergoes hormonal, particularly estrogen, fluctuations.**

2. **Surgically by having your ovaries removed in a procedure called an oopherectomy.**

   - **No ovaries to produce hormones, yet the adrenal glands may create small amounts of estrogen, testosterone, and androstenedione.**
   - **Then aromatase enzymes may convert testosterone and androstenedione hormones into estrogen.**
   - **Perhaps this is why Aromatase Inhibitors seem to work for post-menopausal women because they help stop the aromatase's ability to create estrogen from other hormones.**

3. **Chemically due to chemotherapy.**

   - **Some women can go into temporary menopause and others into permanent menopause due to chemotherapy treatments.**
   - **The closer the woman is to natural menopause when she receives chemotherapy, the more likely she will go into permanent menopause.**

Menopause is the final period. It isn't your final period until you have not had a period for one solid year. It can return after a few months or even up to one year later. In the six to eight months before menopause (the last period), your ovaries produce much less estrogen. Even if your periods are over, your ovaries still produce estrogen and progestin at much lower levels than when you menstruated.

If you have your ovaries removed, your symptoms may be different then if you go into natural menopause. Women who have **one ovary removed** often don't experience a sudden menopause. The remaining ovary continues to produce hormones, and they will more likely go through a natural menopause. Alternatively, a woman who has **both ovaries removed**, a bilateral oopherectomy, may go into menopause immediately with severe symptoms. This is partly why I prolonged finding out if I had a BRCA1 or BRCA2 gene mutation. I didn't want the chance of going right into menopause.

Estrogen decreases in postmenopausal women. Yet, I still don't understand why it is more common for postmenopausal women to get breast cancer than premenopausal women. Reducing estrogen probably decreases breast cancer risk, but it is more likely advanced age and more hormonal fluctuations puts them at a higher risk. Breast cancer is the most common cancer in women, and the risk for it increases with age.

Symptoms of menopause may come on suddenly because of hormonal changes and can last for two to three years. **Try to avoid hormone replacement therapy (HRT).**

HRT increases the risk for breast cancer in many women. Definitely women who have had breast cancer, or those at a greater risk, especially women with the BRCA1 or BRCA2 gene mutation should most likely NOT take HRT.

ALTERNATIVES TO TAKING HORMONE REPLACEMENT THEREAPY (HRT) FOR MENOPAUSE SYMPTOMS:

Avoid things which can trigger hot flashes such as:

- **spicy foods.**
- **caffeine.**
- **hot drinks.**
- **wine or other alcohol.**
- **stress (good luck).**
- **getting overheated (wear cotton and dress in layers).**

- **Know what triggers hot flashes for you and try to avoid them.**
- **Sleep in a cool room with a fan for circulation. Use several thin blankets instead of one heavy one.**
- **Practice deep breathing.**
- **Try aromatherapy by using therapeutic grade oils to smell or put on your body.**
- **Listen to calming music.**
- **Have quality alone time.**
- **Make time for yourself.**

You may also want to try:

- **Seeing an acupuncturist.**
- **Increasing the amount of exercise you do.**
- **Yoga.**
- **Seeing an herbalist regarding vitamin E and an herb called black cohosh (be sure to discuss this with your doctor before taking anything).**

Also, talk to your doctor before adding soy to your diet. Some breast cancer studies suggest soy stimulates estrogen production in the breast. More estrogen in the breast may not be good for women, especially those who have the propensity to produce estrogen-receptor-positive tumors or those with the BRCA1 or BRCA2 gene mutation.

Losing weight may also decrease your menopausal symptoms along with your risk for breast cancer. A good diet with a lot of fresh fruit and vegetables, less red meat, less alcohol, and less junk food can also be helpful.

HORMONE REPLACEMENT THERAPY (HRT) for MENOPAUSAL SYMPTOMS

Breast cancer has interested me for awhile. In writing this book I came across an old file with breast cancer articles I found interesting. I think the side effects of HRT are a very well-kept, yet out in the open, secret which I'd like to further expose.

The article entitled, "My Advice on Estrogen" by Dr. Isadore Rosenfeld came from the weekly Parade section in the Sunday newspaper on October 13, 2002. Dr. Rosenfeld mentions a study which found that the combination of estrogen and progestin taken over many years increases the risk for heart attacks, strokes, breast cancer, and clotting disorders.

Doctors, scientists and the media should be shouting, "DON'T TAKE HORMONE REPLACEMENT THERAPY UNLESS ABSOLUTELY NECESSARY." Doctors should not prescribe HRT for average post-menopausal symptoms, yet I think this is not the case, even in 2010.

I read about a trial by the Women's Health Initiative in which postmenopausal women aged 50 to 79 were given estrogen and progestin, or a placebo, from 1993 to 1998. Interestingly enough, they halted this study early because too many women taking the hormones were getting breast cancer as compared to the placebo group. They determined the health risks of continuing the study, including more women getting **invasive** breast cancer, outweighed the benefit of the study.

In this trial, 16,608 postmenopausal women aged 50-79 were randomly assigned to receive a combination of estrogen and progestin, or a placebo, from the years 1993 to 1998, at 40 clinical centers. The women had screening mammograms and clinical breast exams to establish a baseline, and then they were examined annually.

Their conclusion: **"Relatively short-term combined estrogen plus progestin use increases incident breast cancers, which are diagnosed at a more advanced stage compared with placebo use, and also substantially increases the percentage of women**

with abnormal mammograms. These results suggest estrogen plus progestin may stimulate breast cancer growth and hinder breast cancer diagnosis." As cited in The Journal of American Medical Association (JAMA), Volume 289, No. 24, June 25, 2003 in an article entitled, " The Influence of estrogen plus progestin on breast cancer and mammography in healthy postmenopausal women." "The Women's Health Initiative Randomized Trial." See http://jama.ama-assn.org/cgi/content/abstract/289/24/3243 for more statistics and other related articles.

I am not sure why the use of these hormones would "hinder breast cancer diagnosis" but it makes sense to me that adding hormones into our bodies would increase the risk for breast cancer. My belief is it isn't only the "artificial" hormones which are added to our body, but any hormones, including a woman's own hormonal composition, that makes her more prone to breast cancer when triggered by these supplemental hormones

If a woman has the BRCA1 or BRCA2 gene mutation, or if she has estrogen-receptor-positive breast tissue (meaning breast tissue which is sensitive to estrogen), this can greatly increase her risk for breast cancer when coupled with HRT.

POINTS FROM DR. BARRY:

* **Estrogen receptors are normally found on the breast, brain, kidney, bone, heart, lung, intestine, and prostate.**

I believe we all have cancer cells in our body which lay dormant until something, or a variety of situations, trigger them to multiply and cause trouble. Hormone Replacement Therapy may be one of the triggers, especially in women with breast tissue which is sensitive to estrogen or who have the BRCA1 or BRCA2 gene mutation.

If your breast cancer originates in the lobules, the ends of the milk ducts, then it is referred to as lobular carcinoma. It is thought that most lobular breast cancers are sensitive to hormones. This is important in determining which treatment choice will work best for you. Women who took HRT/hormone replacement therapy and then acquired breast cancer often had it in their lobules instead of in their ducts.

The article entitled, "Breast cancer and hormone-replacement therapy in the million women study." Beral V; Million Women Study Collaborators found in <u>Lancet</u> 2003 Aug 9; 362(9382):419-27 states, "the current use of HRT is associated with an increased risk of incident and fatal breast cancer, the effect is substantially greater for oestrogen-progestagen (other countries outside of the U.S. call estrogen "oestrogen") combinations than for other types of HRT."

- **The Million Women study consisted of 1,084,110 women in the UK who were between the ages of 50 and 64. They conducted it from 1996-2001 in order to determine the effects of HRT on getting breast cancer and also on dying from breast cancer.**
- **Given the enormous size of this study group, one would think the results would be fairly accurate.**
- **Half of the 1,084,110 women (542,055) had used HRT.**
- **Of the women who had taken HRT, 9,364 of them had invasive breast cancer after an average of 2.6 years of follow-up, and 637 women who took HRT died after an average of 4.1 years of follow-up.**
- **It determined that women currently using HRT when they entered the study were more likely than women who had never used HRT to develop breast cancer and die from it. The risk became greatest for women who took oestrogen-progestagen than for women who took other forms of HRT.**

- **In women currently using each type of HRT, the risk for breast cancer increased with the length of time they took them.**
- **10 years of HRT use was estimated to cause 5 additional breast cancers per 1000 women who take only oestrogen, and 19 additional breast cancers per 1000 women who took the combination of oestrogen-progestagen.**
- **It is estimated in the UK that the use of HRT contributed to 20,000 extra women aged 50-64 acquiring breast cancer, in the decade before this study, because of their use of HRT. 15,000 of these women had taken oestrogen-progestagen.**
- **These are significant findings. See <ins>http://www. ncbi.nlm.nih.gov/pubmed/12927427</ins>**

March 26, 2008

I saw a TV commercial by some attorneys seeking women who took hormone replacement therapy and later got breast cancer. I did some internet research and learned that as of March of 2008 more than 5,000 negligence lawsuits have been filed by women across the country against Wyeth Pharmaceuticals, Inc., the maker of Prempro. Prempro is a combination of estrogen and progestin; Premarin is estrogen only. (Premarin is estrogen from a pregnant horse's urine. Some women take it after menopause to help alleviate menopausal symptoms. (Sounds lovely.)

The 5,000 women involved in the lawsuits claim they got breast cancer during or after taking Wyeth's hormones. The drug company even had the nerve to use the fact that they print Prempro's risk for increasing breast cancer on the materials included with the drug for their patients, and for the doctors who prescribe the drug, as a defense against the lawsuits. How many people actually read those little disclaimers?

So their argument seems to be they informed the women and their doctors of the potential, increased risk for breast cancer, and the women took the hormones anyway. I don't hear Wyeth arguing that their hormones don't cause an increased risk of breast cancer, only that they shouldn't be held liable since they gave everyone a warning. Isn't that reassuring! **Most women trust their doctors and the FDA to not give them drugs which can increase their risk for breast cancer and/or give them breast cancer.**

A few of the suits have gone to trial thus far. Three Nevada women and an Arkansas woman were awarded millions of dollars after taking the hormone drugs and then developing breast cancer. Wyeth is appealing the verdicts. Some of the jurors found that Wyeth and Upjohn, a Pfizer unit, showed "reckless disregard" for their products' risks.

Wyeth sold more than $2 billion in hormone replacement drugs prior to the 2002 study by the Women's Health Initiative (WHI) sponsored by the U.S. National Institutes of Health. The study concluded that women who took a combination of estrogen and progestin, as found in Prempro, increased their risk of getting INVASIVE BREAST CANCER SUBSTANTIALLY.

As an attorney I would love to file a suit against Wyeth, with the right attorneys, for the women who acquired breast cancer after taking Premarin or Prempro. I left messages for a few of the attorneys for the women in Nevada and Arkansas, and I never heard back from any of them. Was there a confidential settlement? Is that why we don't hear much about these cases?

I cannot stress enough my belief that women who have had breast cancer, and those at a higher risk should not use HRT/hormone replacement therapy. From my research it appears that the medical community has been aware since at least 1997 that the use of HRT increases the risk of breast cancer.

Were women properly informed of this increased risk of breast cancer from taking estrogen or estrogen/progestin? If they had breast cancer in their family history, did anyone recommend they take the BRCA1 or BRCA2 gene mutation test? If they already had breast cancer, lumps, or biopsies; were they tested for breast tissue sensitivity to estrogen before being put on HRT and given more estrogen? So many questions; not enough answers.

If a woman's lump is estrogen-receptor-positive, then she should not take estrogen. I haven't yet experienced menopause; however, there must be other solutions and treatments to lessen the symptoms of menopause without greatly increasing the risk for breast cancer. (See my "Menopause" section for some ideas.) Is the trade-off of not having hot flashes for potential breast cancer worth it? I don't think so. What about you?

Many doctors no longer recommend hormone replacement therapy (HRT), Hormone Therapy (HT), or Estrogen Therapy (ET) to relieve their patient's menopausal symptoms. You need to think carefully about assuming the risks of taking hormones to help with your menopausal symptoms. Please try other alternatives to decrease them. I encourage you to do your own research on hormones and bio-identical hormones. Talk to your doctor and weigh out the risks and benefits of taking HRT, while considering the length of time that you need to take HRT. Before taking HRT you may want to exhaust all other treatment possibilities for your menopausal symptoms. Then take HRT only if it is absolutely necessary for you to do so.

To summarize, studies agree that women who take HRT increase their risk of getting breast cancer and this potential danger increases with the length of use. The long term use of HRT as estrogen alone, or estrogen plus progestin, has been associated with an increased risk of nonlobular cancer and even more of an increased risk for lobular cancer. The use of estrogen and progestin seems to increase the risk of breast cancer more than the use of estrogen alone. The risk may start decreasing after the HRT is discontinued.

Some studies have determined that women who took HRT and previously had breast cancer experienced a higher rate of recurrence. Most women had the recurrence while taking the HRT.

WEIGHT

Women who are overweight tend to have a higher rate of recurrence of breast cancer than women who aren't. It seems the more fat you have, the more estrogen that can be produced.

Estrogen is a hormone produced by the ovaries, adrenal glands, placenta and fat. Fat creates estrogen. Exercise and eating healthier, meaning, less animal fat, more complex carbohydrates, fruit and vegetables, and a good multi-vitamin can certainly help keep your weight down. Decreasing your weight can decrease your estrogen levels

DIET

The Women's Health Dietary Study was done under the Women's Health Initiative to see if a low fat diet helped decrease the risk of breast cancer. See www.whi.org/findings/dm/dm.php for the findings.

- **48,835 women participated in the study which began in 1993 and ended in March of 2005.**
- **The women ranged in age from 50-79 and were followed for an average of 8.1 years.**

The purpose of the study was to see if a low fat diet (fat making up 20% of the women's calories), combined with a high fruit, vegetable, and grain diet would decrease women's risk of breast cancer and other illnesses. Women in the group which decreased their fat had breast cancer rates 9% lower than the other group which did not decrease their fat.

I think this is a significant reduction; however, the researchers thought this 9% reduction could have been by chance and not due to diet. The researchers concluded a low fat diet may potentially decrease breast cancer risk, especially in women with high fat diets. Again, I think diet is only one contributing factor for breast cancer. Food without hormones and pesticides are likely the best choice. You may want to consider going 'organic'. It is possible that even if you consistently eat healthfully you may still get breast cancer.

Hormones are produced in our bodies and from external forces such as the foods we eat. Hormones in foods can't be good for us. Personally, I have decreased my meat intake. When I eat meat I choose the kind without hormones. I also look for food without additives and hormones. It is best to be as natural as possible with what we put into our bodies. This means less frozen and manufactured food; more fresh fruits and vegetables (organic, when possible). What I have refused to give up is my daily chocolate. For me it is medicinal.

Decreasing animal fat and calories should help to decrease the risk of getting breast cancer. Women with high fat diets may have more estrogen in their blood than women with lower fat diets. Thus, a low fat diet may be better for you than a high fat diet if you want to reduce your risk. A diet filled with complex carbohydrates and fiber is probably better than a high fat diet.

Consuming five to nine servings of fruit or vegetables per day is thought to be cancer-fighting. Also, if you fill up on fruits and vegetables, then you won't eat as much fat or sweets. I know it is a lot to ask and some sacrifices must be made; yet isn't your life worth it?

It is believed that vegetables from the cabbage family considered *cruciferous vegetables* have high amounts of natural cancer-fighting phytochemicals (unique chemicals found in plants). The vegetables in this group include: broccoli, brussel sprouts, cabbage (especially Savoy cabbage), cauliflower, horseradish, and radishes.

Fruits and vegetables are great sources of antioxidants and may give the body some needed protective enzymes. You may want to read a book called How to Reduce Your Risk of Breast Cancer by Jon Michnovicz, M.D., PH.D and Diane S. Klein, copyrighted in 1994, for more information on how a healthy diet can help reduce your risk. You may want to do some of your own research as there are many helpful books out there.

To reiterate, I think your life can only be enhanced by increasing your intake of fruits and vegetables, especially if they are organic, along with decreasing junk food, fried foods and any animal fat you eat. In addition to ingesting helpful plant chemicals into your body; eating more fruit and vegetables may help keep your weight down.

EXCERCISE

Exercising five days a week is optimal yet strive for a minimum of three days a week. Exercise decreases stress, keeps us closer to a "normal" body weight, reduces fat, and seems to affect our hormones in positive ways. Thus, regular exercise is said to decrease the risk of getting breast cancer.

ALCOHOL

Drinking more than two drinks of alcohol a day can also contribute to whether you will get breast cancer. There is a connection between increased alcohol consumption and an increase in production of estrogen. For some women, additional estrogen can directly contribute to their getting breast cancer.

ENVIRONMENT

While at the San Diego airport before our trip to Italy, I sat next to a man who had been here on a conference. I don't remember his exact profession yet it had something to do with mapping out the areas where certain illnesses occur at a higher rate than in other communities. Although I didn't mention my recent breast cancer diagnosis, he told me about areas in the East coast that have very high incidences of breast cancer. I think he mentioned Long Island, New York (perhaps because there are a lot of Ashkenazi Jewish women there) as one of the places with a high rate. He also shared that pesticide may contribute to breast cancer. It is best to live in an environment as free of chemicals as possible. You may want to choose cleaners for your home that have less chemicals and are more organic.

Andrea Schneider

GENETICS-THE BRCA1 AND BRCA2 GENE MUTATION

A few weeks after meeting with the ob-gyn to discuss ovarian cancer and the BRCA1 and BRCA2 gene mutation test, I received a notice that if I wanted to meet with the gene counselor, I must call for an appointment within the next two weeks. I procrastinated and then finally scheduled it. Mom, my daughter, Gabby, and my young son, Andrew, met with genetics counselor Tammy on August 27, 2007. She asked us questions about our family tree on my mom's and dad's sides. She asked about family history regarding all types of cancers, and specifically wanted to know about melanomas, ovarian, pancreatic, colon and breast cancers.

In my research about the BRCA1 and BRCA2 gene mutation, I found out the following:

A man with the BRCA1 mutation has a higher risk for prostate and breast cancer than men without it. A woman with the BRCA1 gene mutation has a greater risk of breast cancer in both of her breasts as well as ovarian cancer, than women who do not have this gene mutation. People who have the gene mutation have a greater risk for colon cancer thus a regular colonoscopy is necessary.

Men with a BRCA2 mutation have an increased risk for breast, prostate, and pancreatic cancer. Women with the BRCA2 mutation have a greater risk for breast cancer and an increased risk of ovarian cancer. They have a reduced risk for ovarian cancer compared to a woman with the BRCA1 mutation.

A woman with a BRCA mutation has between a 56 and 87% risk for breast cancer in her lifetime.

If you have either the BRCA1 or BRCA2 gene mutation, then every cell in your body has that gene mutation. BRCA1 and BRCA2 genes help check on and repair DNA. They help fight off cancer and other illnesses. Since the genes are mutated, they may not be able to work to their full capacity. Thus, they can't do their job to ward off illnesses nor protect you when you are exposed to whatever may cause breast cancer. Also, with this mutation your body may be more

138

sensitive to hormones like estrogen and progestin, a high fat diet, alcohol, and other factors which contribute to breast cancer.

POINTS FROM DR. BARRY:

- **BRCA proteins are involved in the repairing of damaged DNA.**
- **When BRCA is damaged then the faulty BRCA protein does not repair DNA as well as a non-damaged BRCA protein would do.**

Before you are tested for the BRCA1 or BRCA2 mutation you need genetic counseling to be fully aware of the risks and benefits associated with the test and how to handle the information you receive. If you know you are someone who won't do anything with the information, then don't waste your time or money taking the test.

POINTS FROM DR. BARRY:

- **Whether you are negative or positive for the gene mutation may be useful for your children to know.**

Gene counseling can be helpful if you have many people in your family (especially first degree relatives - mother, daughter, sister) who have had either breast or ovarian cancer. Even without this strong family history, if you are diagnosed with breast cancer (especially before the age of 50), then you may want genetic counseling and the test to help you decide if you want to choose a bilateral mastectomy and/or an oopherectomy (removal of ovaries) for treatment and/or prevention. If you do have the BRCA1 or BRCA2 gene mutation, then a bilateral mastectomy may be your best treatment choice.

If you have the BRCA1 or BRCA2 gene mutation, **then removing your OVARIES** between the age of 35 and 50 decreases the risk for ovarian cancer by as much as 97% and **reduces your risk for**

BREAST cancer by 47-61%. If you do this after age 50, it decreases the risk for ovarian cancer by as much as 89% and breast cancer by about 48%.

MASTECTOMIES decrease the risk of a mutation carrier getting breast cancer by as much as 90-95%. Women who have either the BRCA1 or BRCA2 gene mutation and have an oopherectomy (removal of ovaries), and then take Tamoxifen or have a bilateral mastectomy and oopherectomy by the age of 30, may have **survival rates similar to women who do not have the genetic mutation**.

There may be differences in the way breastfeeding and pregnancy affect a woman who has a BRCA1 or BRCA2 mutation as compared to a woman who does not have it.

The BRCA1 and BRCA2 mutations can't be taken lightly. If you have either one, it is best to find out early and take the necessary steps to decrease your chances for ovarian and breast cancer. Talk to your doctor about your personal risk factors if you have either gene mutation, and specifically ask how each treatment choice will decrease your risk for breast and ovarian cancer.

Tammy, the genetics counselor, shared the following **Statistics:**

- **60% of breast cancer is sporadic, by chance.**
- **30% of breast cancer is familial (possibly the whole family had been exposed to something, yet no one is sure what).**
- **10% of breast cancer is genetic and due to the gene mutation of BRCA1 or BRCA2.**
- **If you have the BRCA2 gene mutation you have a higher risk of melanoma.**
- **The average female has a 1 in 8 (12.5%) risk for breast cancer by the age of 70.**
- **A female with the gene mutation may have up to an 87% risk for breast cancer.**

Tammy gave me a brochure called "Hereditary Breast and Ovarian Cancer Syndrome-A Patient's Guide to Risk Assessment" (the brochure is from Myriad Genetic Laboratories, they are the company that does the BRCA gene testing).

According to the Myriad brochure, **the personal and family history which is considered for whether you may be at risk for having a BRCA gene mutation is:**

- **Breast cancer before the age of 50.**
- **Ovarian cancer at any age.**
- **Male breast cancer at any age.**
- **Bilateral breast cancer.**
- **Both breast and ovarian cancer.**
- **Relative with a BRCA mutation.**
- **Ashkenazi/Eastern European Jewish descent.**

I don't know which of the above factors, if any, has more weight in calculating your risk. It seems you are at more risk to have the gene if you have breast cancer before age 50. Unfortunately, 12% of the female population is expected to have breast cancer during their lifetime and the odds go up as we age.

According to the Myriad brochure:

"In some families we see more cancer than we would expect by chance alone. Determining which of these families have cancer related to an inherited gene mutation is important, as the cancer risks in hereditary cancer families are much higher than the general population. Hereditary breast and ovarian cancer syndrome is an inherited condition that causes an increased risk of ovarian cancer and early onset breast cancer (often before the age of 50)." (I was 41 when mine was diagnosed.) "The vast majority of hereditary breast and ovarian cancer is due to an alteration or mutation in either the BRCA1 or BRCA2 genes. These mutations can be inherited from either your mother of father."

The Myriad brochure states that these are the **"Cancer risks for BRCA gene mutation carriers"**:

- **Women who have the BRCA mutation have a 56-87% risk of getting breast cancer as compared to 8% for the general population.**
- **Women who have the BRCA mutation have a 27-44% risk of ovarian cancer as compared to less than 1% for the general population.**
- **Women who have the BRCA mutation have a 48-64% risk of getting a secondary primary breast cancer as compared to 2-11% for the general population.**
- **Men who have the BRCA mutation have a 6% risk of breast cancer as compared to less than .05% for the general population**

If these statistics are available, why isn't this information shared aggressively with the general public? This frustrates me. When a woman is diagnosed with breast cancer, perhaps a discussion regarding the gene test should take place. This would definitely help with her decision making. If you have a BRCA mutation, why would you want to run the risk of a 48-64% chance of getting breast cancer again? Further, you'll worry that your cancer may go undetected before it spreads to other parts of your body.

The Myriad brochure discusses **"Managing hereditary breast and ovarian cancer risk."**

- **It recommends increased surveillance for women with a hereditary disposition toward breast and ovarian cancer.**
- **At 18 to 21, they should begin monthly self breast exams and annual or semiannual clinical breast exams (a breast exam by a doctor) starting at ages 25 to 35.**

- **They should have yearly mammograms and/or a MRI beginning between the ages of 25 to 35.**
- **An annual or semiannual transvaginal ultrasound and testing for CA-125 to screen for ovarian cancer beginning between the ages of 25 and 35.**

I don't know why they mention these age spans. It would seem most prudent to begin at the earliest age possible to get an early baseline to compare future tests to. Of course, you must have the best health insurance, disability insurance, and life insurance possible before you are diagnosed with the gene mutation, breast, or ovarian cancer.

The brochure also discusses **"Chemoprevention."**

- **Drugs such as Tamoxifen have been shown to reduce the risk of breast cancer in high risk women.**
- **Oral contraceptives may reduce the risk of ovarian cancer in women with BRCA1 or BRCA2 mutations. (Perhaps by altering the hormone cycle.)**

"Preventive Surgery" is also discussed in the brochure.

- **Preventive mastectomy significantly reduces the risk of breast cancer in women with BRCA1 or BRCA2 mutations.**
- **Preventive removal of the ovaries significantly reduces the risk of ovarian cancer, and also decreases the risk of breast cancer, in women with BRCA1 or BRCA2 mutations.**

According to Tammy, the genetics counselor I saw, if you take the blood test (now the test can be done with saliva) and they determine you have a gene mutation, then a bilateral mastectomy and ovarian screening, and possibly removal of your ovaries may be recommended. She indicated that a transvaginal ultrasound is the best screening tool for ovarian cancer. (Ask your doctor about this test.) If you remove your ovaries you decrease, but do not totally eliminate your chance for ovarian cancer. If you have your ovaries removed during premenopause, it will accelerate your menopause. You also won't be able to get pregnant.

I found out in 2010 that you can now take this gene test by spitting into a cup and don't have to give blood. Your choice which way you want to do the test. You should be able to discuss the gene test with your ob/gyn or regular doctor. They can help you determine if you should take the test. You may be able to take it right in their office. If needed, they can refer you to a geneticist.

The Myriad brochure has a chart entitled, **"proactive cancer management reduces the risks."** It lists the **following preventive measures** along with the **percentages** of risk reduction regarding ovarian and breast cancer.

- **Tamoxifen reduces (it doesn't indicate when to start taking it) the risk of breast cancer by 53%.**
- **Mastectomy reduces the risk of breast cancer by 90% or more. (My doctors told me that my bilateral mastectomy reduced my risk by 98-100%. Your risk reduction will depend on the type of breast cancer you have and your risk factors.)**
- **Oophorectomy (I didn't know that having your ovaries out is called an oophorectomy until I met with the genetic counselor Tammy.) reduces the risk of breast cancer by up to 68% and ovarian cancer by up to 96%. (Wow!)**
- **Oral contraceptives reduce the risk of ovarian cancer by up to 60%.**

I am not sure if these statistics refer to your personal risk. It is difficult to give across the board statistics for everyone. Talk to your doctor about your risks.

POINTS FROM DR. BARRY:

- **The above are statistics. They look at groups of people and compare them.**

Reading the gene mutation brochure was upsetting to me. I am upset that removing a woman's ovaries and breasts may still be the best options for decreasing her risk of ovarian and breast cancer. I am upset that this data is not being discussed more. Maybe it is being discussed and public knowledge, but I haven't come across it before. Have you?

I never had imagined removing one's ovaries could decrease the risk for breast cancer until doing my research for this book. I guess that makes sense because whether you get breast cancer must have something to do with your personal hormones. I learned that the ovaries are the main source of a premenopausal woman's estrogen production. As I've discussed numerous times, estrogen levels can be an indicator of whether you will get breast cancer. The doctors never discussed this with me. How does this all fit together? I'm still wondering. What about you?

One morning while cuddling in bed with Gabby, almost 11-years-old at the time, I told her I'd do my best to find answers to breast cancer before she is old enough to face this possibility. I hope as you read this, you will think of some way to improve the diagnosis, treatment, and prevention of breast cancer.

The gene mutation brochure mentions there are "**Three types of tests to look for the BRCA1 and BRCA2 mutations.**

- **The comprehensive BRCAnalysis: Full sequence and large rearrangement analysis of BRCA1 and BRCA2.**

- **Single site BRCAnalysis: mutation-specific analysis is done for individuals with a known BRCA1 or BRCA2 mutation in their family.**
- **Multisite 3 BRCAnalysis which analyzes the three most common BRCA1 and BRCA2 mutations in people of Ashkenazi (family heritage is Jewish from Eastern Europe) ancestry.**

Tammy said with Ashkenazi Jewish people they analyze the BRCA1 gene for two possible changes to the gene. (According to the brochure, they specifically examine the 187delAG and 5385insC sites on the BRCA1 gene. (Although this is code which only geneticists, scientists, and doctors can relate to, if you are of Ashkenazi Jewish descent, you will want to be aware of this.) Then they look at the BRCA2 gene for one change to the gene (the 6174delT site). What does this mean? If they don't find changes/mutations to either of those genes, then they go to a wider spectrum of gene testing. If you are not of Jewish Askenazi descent, then they start your analysis differently.

POINTS FROM DR. BARRY:

A "gene" is a piece of DNA, and DNA is made up of long strands of G's, T's, A's and C's

T=Thymidine

G=Guanine

A=Adenine

C=Cytosine

Del=deletion

Ins=insertion

The number refers to where along the gene the change is.

According to the Myriad brochure, the BRCA1 and BRCA2 mutations may be passed on in a family. If you have a mutation for either of these genes, your parents, your children, and your siblings have up to a 50% chance of having the same gene mutation. Other relatives may also have the gene mutation.

Tammy stated the results of the blood test are accurate, and the test is the only way to identify whether you have the gene mutation. If you get a positive result, meaning you have the mutation, you are at a higher risk for both breast cancer and ovarian cancer. If you get a negative result, meaning the gene test does not show a mutation, and you have already had breast cancer, then they won't know what caused the cancer. If they get an "uncertain" result this means there is a gene change, but they don't know what the significance of the change is. This is treated as a negative result and more results would need to be gathered from other people with similar gene changes to see if these people develop cancer before conclusions can be drawn about the significance of the gene change.

The brochure explains there are several "**Possible test results**:

- **A positive result means you are at an increased risk for ovarian and/or breast cancer; therefore, you must talk with your doctor about his/her recommendations for mutation carriers.**
- **A negative result with a BRCA1 or BRCA2 gene mutation previously identified in your family means you have no increased breast or ovarian cancer risk. Base your medical cancer screening on the general population cancer screening recommendations (and perhaps your personal and family history of cancer).**
- **A negative result with no mutation previously identified in your family significantly reduces your risk for hereditary breast or ovarian cancer. Base your medical cancer screening on**

your negative test results and your personal and family history of cancer.
- **An uncertain variant means your cancer risk is not fully defined. (They don't know enough about that specific gene change to know if it will cause cancer.) Base your cancer management on your personal and family history of cancer.**

- **POINTS FROM DR. BARRY:**
- **An uncertain variant means there is still a lot we don't know. Kind of like who killed Nicole Simpson - we think we know but...**
- **There is a lot of information that we don't fully understand or know what to do with yet.**

You may prefer not to have the gene test done. This is certainly your option. You must consider what actions, if any, you are willing to take if the information comes back positive, meaning you have the BRCA1 or BRCA2 gene mutation. Will this information prey on your mind and create more worry? Will you be proactive? If you are not willing to take proactive cancer management; Tamoxifen, Mastectomy, Oophorectomy, or oral contraception, then it may be best for you not to take this test.

I had heard that a positive result indicating a gene mutation can effect your ability to get health, life and disability insurance. I have been told by a doctor friend that this is an important misconception. She says there are multiple state and Federal laws to prevent discrimination because of genetics. You can do your own research on this topic. Of course, a result indicating no gene mutation will lessen any concern you may have about whether or not you and your family have this gene mutation. It can also alleviate any fear that you are at a higher risk for breast and ovarian cancer, as compared to the general population.

August 28, 2008

I had my breasts removed on September 5, 2006. I originally saw Tammy, the genetic counselor, on August 27, 2007 and got the approval to have the gene test. I just wasn't in a rush to take this test. I didn't want to have my ovaries removed if it came back positive for the gene mutation. On August 12, 2008 I finally got the courage to have the blood test. Tammy called me on August 25, 2008 to tell me she had the results. I had to come in to meet with her to receive them. She does not even open the results until the patient is in her office. I went to see Tammy on August 28, 2008, almost one year to-the-date since my first meeting with Tammy. Tammy had two envelopes from Myriad. One indicated they had tested my blood for the gene mutation often found in Ashkenazi Jewish women and I tested negative for the mutation. The next envelope checked my blood for the gene mutation with regard to the population at large. Thankfully this one turned out to be negative for that mutation as well. I felt enormous relief, as did my ovaries, my mother, and my daughter.

INTERPLAY OF the ABOVE RISK FACTORS:

I believe all of the ABOVE factors interplay and thus, there is probably not one reason women get breast cancer. This makes it challenging for researchers to figure out THE cause of breast cancer. I am sure finding the cause would help us find a cure, yet we may be able to discover the cure without knowing why women get breast cancer.

There are many heavy men who drink alcohol, consume a fatty diet, have been exposed to environmental carcinogens; and yet men rarely get breast cancer.

POINTS FROM DR. BARRY:

- **There are plenty of overweight women who never get breast cancer. This is a complex issue.**

What is the biggest difference between men and women? It would seem to be our genetic and hormonal composition. These other factors I have mentioned may be stimulants or minor factors, but the primary reason women get breast cancer, in my opinion, is due to our genes and hormones and the fact that they are women.

It is not one thing that causes breast cancer and it may be different things in different women. Perhaps a group of women are exposed to the same factors, yet only some of them acquire breast cancer. Similar to when everyone in your family is exposed to the flu but not everyone gets sick. Some people have stronger immune systems so they may not be as sensitive to germs, viruses, or risk factors.

Since there are so many factors which contribute to breast cancer, it is not easy to determine what "causes it."

POINTS FROM DR. BARRY:

- **This is called the "multi-hit" hypothesis of cancer.**

Some people always get a cold, and others who are exposed to cold or flu viruses never get sick. Why? Maybe some people are more susceptible to certain illnesses than others.

POINTS FROM DR. BARRY:

- **It is possible that some people are more susceptible to illnesses than others.**
- **Habits such as not frequently washing one's hands and then touching the nose or mouth may cause someone to inoculate themselves with a cold or flu.**

Clearly in the case of breast cancer, women are much more susceptible to getting breast cancer than men. Why is that? The major difference is that we are WOMEN, and we have a different hormonal composition than men.

POINTS FROM DR. BARRY:

- **Women's breasts are more developed, functional and more hormonal than men's breasts.**

I am not suggesting a woman causes her breast cancer; however, she can take action to help prevent it. If she is diagnosed with it, then she can try to avoid a recurrence through preventive measures. This needs to become a way of life. To derive any benefits, it cannot be once in awhile activities."

PREVENTION/THINGS YOU CAN CONTROL:

- **It is important to have a diet high in fruit and vegetables, whole grains, while low in animal fat and processed food. Try eating fewer things that come in wrappers.**
- **Tomatoes and vegetables from the *cruciferous* (broccoli, cauliflower, brussel sprouts...) family may decrease breast cancer risks so eat plenty of these.**
- **A lower fat diet is said to decrease the risk of a recurrence of breast cancer.**
- **A good multivitamin with folic acid may also be helpful.**
- **Not being overweight.**
- **Have your first baby before the age of 35.**
- **Breastfeed (although breastfeeding and pregnancy may have a negative effect if you have a BRCA1 or BRCA2 gene mutation or have breast tissue that is estrogen- receptor-positive.)**
- **DO NOT take hormone therapy namely estrogen, or estrogen and progestin at menopause, especially if you are at a higher risk for getting breast cancer.**

- **Talk to your doctor about the increased risk of taking fertility drugs to get pregnant. Make an informed decision based on the risks and benefits.**
- **Drink less than two glasses of alcohol a day.**
- **Do self-exams and get anything suspicious checked right away.**
- **Have mammograms on a regular basis.**
- **Be an assertive advocate for your own well-being.**
- **Exercising five days a week is optimal, yet aim for a minimum of three days a week. This decreases stress levels, keeps us closer to our "normal" body weight, reduces fat, and probably affects our hormones. Thus, regular exercise is thought to decrease the risk for breast cancer.**
- **The other factors mentioned before come into play, yet your own hormones could very well be the final determinant of whether you will get breast cancer.**
- **The BRCA1 or BRCA2 gene mutation is a major factor, if you have it.**

MY RISK FACTORS:

ALCOHOL/OBESITY/CAFFEINE

I did whatever I could to decrease my risk for breast cancer. I don't smoke and never have. I have exercised since age 18, not always regularly yet enough to stay in fairly good shape. I am nearly 5'6". When I became pregnant with Gabby I weighed 119 pounds. I gained 46 pounds with her so I grew to 165 pounds. I never lost 10 of those pounds. When I became pregnant with Andrew at age 39, I weighed 129 pounds and wore a size 6 or 8. I added another 42 pounds with him. Within 6 months of his birth, I returned to 137 pounds. Now at the age of 45, I am 129 pounds. Thus, I've managed my weight fairly well and certainly have never been obese.

I have rarely had alcohol since getting pregnant with Gabby in 1996. I may drink four or five times per year and only a few alcoholic beverages. I may have three cups of coffee a year and very few sodas. I don't always eat enough fruit or vegetables, but I am working on it. Making smoothies in my blender allows me to have a lot of fruit. I might not always eat enough fruit and vegetables, but, I do eat chocolate almost every day of my life. Fortunately, it is rich in antioxidants.

ETHNICITY

A factor I have no control over is my genetic background. I am of Ashkenazi, Eastern European, Jewish descent. For some reason, Jewish women from Eastern European descent have a higher risk for breast cancer and for having the BRCA1 or BRCA2 gene mutation than other women. Although no one knows why this is, it may be due to there not being much intermarriage, until recently. With a tighter gene pool, the mutation could stay within it.

FAMILY HISTORY

My oldest brother had melanomas removed from his back several years ago, and he is fine. My father had prostate cancer in his late 60's and then died at 74 from a large, cancerous tumor attached to his kidney and all of his internal organs. He died two weeks after his diagnosis. His cancer probably has no bearing on my breast cancer, but my brother's melanoma may be related making it more likely we have the BRCA1 or BRCA2 gene mutations. As I've mentioned, once I had the courage to take the test, I found out that I'm not a carrier of the BRCA1 or BRCA2 gene mutation. I could sleep better at night.

You may also have a higher risk of breast cancer if your mother, daughter, or sister had breast cancer. I do not have any sisters, and my mother, who is now 76, had several benign lumps removed but never had breast cancer. Her mother, my maternal grandmother, had a mastectomy in her 70's. Back then they essentially chopped off one's breast. Grandma Syl chose not to have reconstruction, and often showed all of us her lack of breast and her prosthesis.

Unfortunately, we can't really know what someone is going through or feeling until we walk a similar path. Thinking about my grandma making it through her more radical mastectomy gave me support and encouragement. If she could recover at a much later age, I certainly could while still young and strong. Grandma died at the age of 89 after a stroke. She never had a recurrence of breast cancer. In her 80's she told me she never had breast cancer. I never figured that out. Was her age and dementia responsible for her not remembering she had breast cancer; or did they make a mistake about her having cancer after they removed her breast and discovered this? Did she have early stage breast cancer like mine and then later was told it really wasn't cancer. Some deem DCIS as "pre-cancer." In any case she never had breast cancer again, and she didn't die from it.

STRESS and LACK OF SLEEP

A primary factor which most likely contributes to breast cancer and many illnesses is stress. I have always thought I handle stress well, at least on the outside, but I probably internalize it. Going to law school, and then studying for the bar exam, were stressful. Being an attorney was demanding. Losing my dad in April of 2003 and then having my mom move in with us had me on edge. Then I changed careers, completed a major remodel on my house by adding on 1400 square feet and totally redid the older section of our home, while pregnant. I felt fine outwardly overall, but I have no idea what may have been going on inside of my body with all of that turmoil.

As a mom with a professional career, who works from the house, it is often tough to balance quantity time versus quality time with my kids. I find it stressful to accomplish my business work while also entertaining young children. It is definitely a balancing act and can be very taxing to "do it all." I certainly appreciate the struggles my parents had making a living and raising children, more now as a mother than I did before having them.

We may all carry some form of cancer cells inside us, and they don't show their vile selves until our immune systems are weaker. Unfortunately, stress is a fact of life for all of us. We must learn ways to both control and decrease it. Exercise, especially yoga, has been helpful for me in alleviating stress.

Lack of sleep also contributes to getting sick. Being pregnant and then nursing in the night, I hadn't slept a full seven hours without interruption in over two and a half years. With my older child, Gabby, I didn't sleep well during my pregnancy. Then she didn't sleep through the night until four years old. And if she didn't sleep through the night - I didn't either.

When our resistance is down, illness can take over. Outwardly I looked healthy but we don't know what is happening inside of our bodies.

ENVIRONMENT

Remember that guy I met in the airport, his studies indicated pesticides may contribute to breast cancer. I grew up in Illinois next to a cornfield. The farmer used pesticides. They fumigated with a lot of bug sprays in the summers. No one really knows yet what causes breast cancer. Sometimes I'm not even sure if the experts do either. I think it is important to keep exploring all of these variables.

ESTROGEN AND PROGESTERONE USE (hormone replacement therapy)

I have not used either of these. I never took fertility drugs.

EARLY MENSTRUATION

I started my period at 14. At 41 I became diagnosed with breast cancer. So, I had a period for 27 years by then. This isn't a long time in terms of an increased risk factor for breast cancer.

Having a period for 40 years or more may increase your risk of getting breast cancer due to the length of hormone fluctuations.

HIGH FAT DIET

Besides eating about an ounce of chocolate every day, I eat healthfully. I avoid fried foods, try to eat a salad every day, along with some fruits and vegetables. I rarely eat a red meat or much dairy. I have nuts every day and do my best to drink eight glasses of water each day. Growing up in the Midwest, we had meat for dinner almost every night.

POINTS FROM DR. BARRY:

- **Nuts are high in fat but it is doubtful they would contribute to getting DCIS.**

NOT HAVING A CHILD OR HAVING A CHILD AFTER THE AGE of 35

I had one child at 32 and the other at 40. So, I may be at a wash here.

POSTMENOPAUSAL WOMEN

Most breast cancer occurs after the age of 50. They discovered mine at 41. I am not menopausal yet.

Bottom line, the healthier our lifestyle the better off we are. There are many factors which contribute to whether we will be diagnosed with breast cancer or other illnesses. We can control some factors, others we cannot. We have no power over our genetic dispositions to illnesses. Hopefully, gene therapy and research will change this soon.

C. BREAST CANCER SCREENING

NORMAL SCREENING: A QUICK GAMEPLAN

- Do your breast self-examination at least once a month.
- Get a physical examination by a licensed health care provider such as a surgeon, primary care physician, gynecologist, nurse practitioner, or other medical provider who has extensive experience with breasts, at least once a year. Do this more often if you have something suspicious, are at higher risk for getting breast cancer, or have had breast cancer.
- Get a baseline mammogram and a yearly exam unless a more frequent one is necessary.
- Consider getting the nipple aspiration fluid (NAF) test once a year. (See information about this later in this section.)
- If you have a family history of melanomas, breast, ovarian, or colon cancer then think about scheduling genetic counseling and taking the test for the BRCA1 or BRCA2 gene mutation to determine if you have either gene mutation.
- If you have the BRCA1 or BRCA2 gene mutation your chances of getting breast and ovarian cancer are much higher.
- If you have the gene mutation, consider having prophylactic mastectomies. (This means you do not have breast cancer, yet prefer to substantially cut your risk for breast cancer by removing your breasts.)
- Depending on your risk, your age, and whether you still want to birth a child, consider having

**an oopherectomy (removal of your ovaries), if
you have the BRCA1 or BRCA2 gene mutation.**
- **An oopherectomy accelerates menopause so
you won't be able to get pregnant. You will
substantially lower your risk for ovarian cancer
and greatly reduce your risk for breast cancer, if
you have the BRCA1 or BRCA2 gene mutation.**
- **Get anything suspicious checked immediately.
Do your homework and be assertive about
getting the appropriate tests for your situation.**

SCREENING TESTS

BRCA1 OR BRCA2 GENE MUTATION TEST

Before you get tested for the BRCA1 or BRCA2 mutation you
must have genetic counseling. You must know the risks and benefits
of having the test and what to do with the information you might
receive. If you won't do anything with the information then don't
take the test.

You should have **genetic counseling** if there are many people in
your family (especially first-degree relatives-mother, daughter, sister)
who had either breast or ovarian cancer. Even without a strong family
history, if you are diagnosed with breast cancer (especially before
age 50), then genetic counseling can be helpful with your decision
to choose a bilateral mastectomy and/or an oopherectomy (removal
of your ovaries) for treatment and/or prevention. If you do have the
BRCA1 or BRCA2 gene mutation, then a bilateral mastectomy and/
or and oopherectomy may be your best treatments choices.

See my previous, lengthy discussion of the gene test and the
BRCA1 and BRCA2 gene mutation in my section entitled, "**Breast
Cancer Screening: Genetics-The BRCA1 and BRCA2 Gene
Mutation** starting on page 138."

HALO NAF

The HALO NAF Breast PAP test can allegedly detect **early abnormal breast cancer cells possibly 7 or 8 years before a mammogram can detect a lump.** (Mammograms don't look at cells.) Thus, the HALO NAF test may be able to find abnormal cells during their pre-invasive stages.

The five minute test is done in the doctor's office. Suction cups, like breast pumps used during breastfeeding, are attached to each breast; the breast is compressed; and light suction is applied to bring nipple fluid to the surface. The fluid is collected and sent to the laboratory for analysis.

According to the literature I received about the test, "Since almost all breast cancer starts in the milk ducts, the best way to analyze early signs of breast health changes is by examining nipple aspirate fluid (NAF) from these ducts. Just as a Pap smear shows if you are at risk for cervical cancer, the HALO System helps determine who is at higher risk for breast cancer by alerting your physician to abnormal cells that might develop into breast cancer years from now."

If most breast cancer starts out in the milk ducts and you remove your milk ducts via a mastectomy, one could presume there would be only a slight chance for breast cancer. Although I am not suggesting every woman have a mastectomy, facts like this helped me make my decision to have a bilateral mastectomy.

The Halo breast cancer risk assessment **does not replace a mammogram,** but the literature suggests it be used as a **supplement to a mammogram**. The mammogram screens for the presence of LUMPS and abnormal looking areas versus the HALO NAF test which takes fluid out of the breast(s) to be analyzed for ABNORMAL CELLS.

It makes sense that finding abnormal CELLS before they have grown into an abnormal LUMP would be beneficial. The literature also encourages women from ages 20-59 to take the HALO breast cancer risk assessment test.

Most women don't start with mammograms until age 40. The HALO NAF test could be especially helpful for young women who are often not good candidates for mammograms because of their dense breast tissue.

In the literature Dr. Baxter-Jones is quoted,, "the test determines if the cells are normal, pre-malignant or cancerous. Depending on the results and the woman's family history and risk factors, we can determine the best treatment plan in collaboration with surgeons, oncologists and other specialists. This test is beneficial to all women because it provides a way to routinely evaluate and manage breast health which can lead to an early diagnosis of breast cancer, It is especially helpful for younger women who are not recommended for mammography and for those with dense breasts, where mammography may not provide a clear image." She recommends women have the NAF screening test as a baseline starting at age 25.

I read in the literature that Dr. Baxter-Jones, M.D., M.B.A, a board-certified obstetrician/gynecologist lived not too far from my home. She is recognized as the first physician in the country to use this FDA approved test. I called her office to find out more about the test. I learned the test costs $95. If fluid is produced, then it gets analyzed for an additional $45. I do not think insurance covers this test.

I would have had it but I was told I could not get the test until three to six months after breastfeeding, preferably six months. I didn't want to delay my mastectomies for this test, although I wondered if it would find abnormal cells in my breasts. Looking back I wish I had discussed this with Dr. Baxter-Jones, even though I had recently been breastfeeding. Since my breasts would be removed soon, the HALO NAF results could have been easily compared to what they found in my breasts when they analyzed them after my mastectomies.

Please see the websites www.paptestforthebreast.com and www. neomatrix.com for more information on the HALO-NAF test. This test may not be available in your area yet.

It is thought all or most breast cancer begins in the milk ducts. Thus, it would seem early testing of the cells in the ducts makes clear sense. A baseline of what your cells look like during the first test can be compared to later evaluations. Like a mammogram, this test can be done every year to detect any changes.

Testing Nipple Aspiration Fluid (NAF) is not a new concept. The inventor of the cervical Pap smear, George Papanicolaou, talked about getting fluid out of the milk ducts by using suction on the nipples back in the 1950's. The fluid which comes out of the ducts is not milk but nipple aspiration fluid or NAF. Several studies on NAF were done in the 1970's.

A study by Margaret Wrensch, Eileen King, Nicholas Petrakis and many others, did testing on **2701 volunteer women in the San Francisco area from 1973-1980.**

- The women were between 25 and 54 years old at the time of fluid testing.
- Follow-up for 87% of these women or 2,343 of the original 2,701 women, with an average of 12.7 years of follow-up took place.

POINTS FROM DR. BARRY:

- **The follow-up of 12.7 years may be too short.**
- **Some breast cancer survivors get a recurrence as much as 20 years later.**

- 4.4% of the 2,343 women or 104 women developed breast cancer. The scientists compared what had actually happened to the women, over time, in terms of getting breast cancer to their initial fluid evaluation years earlier.
- Scientists determined if **no fluid** came out of the woman's breast, she had the lowest risk for breast cancer. 352 of the original women tested produced no fluid and, 9 of the 352, which is 2.6%, later developed breast cancer.

- In the group of women with **fluid and normal cells,** their risk for breast cancer grew. 56 of the 1,291 women, which is 4.3%, fell into this category and later became diagnosed with breast cancer.
- In the group of women with **fluid and cells with epithelial hyperplasia,** 18 of the 327 women, which is 5.5%, later developed breast cancer.
- In the group of women with fluid **and cells with atypical hyperplasia,** 6 of the 58 women, which is 10.3%, later acquired breast cancer.
- The scientists determined that women with **atypical hyperplasia who had first-degree relatives** with breast cancer were more likely to get breast cancer than those without a family history of breast cancer.

POINTS FROM DR. BARRY:

- **The above results are confusing since the incidence of breast cancer in the general population is 12%.**
- **Was the sample size of 2,343 women large enough?**
- **If you had the NAF test and produced no fluid was your risk 2.6% or 12%?**
- **If you had the NAF test and had atypical hyperplasia was your risk 10.3% or 12% and is the difference statistically significant?**

It is interesting that extensive research has been done on NAF, nipple aspiration fluid, but it is not widely accepted as a screening method for early stage breast cancer. I anticipate this will change. It seems women would have a stronger chance of surviving breast cancer if the cancer or "pre-cancer" could be discovered in the **CELL** stage before it becomes a cancerous lump.

To reiterate, in the Wrensch/King/Petrakis study, the increase in breast cancer moved along the spectrum of normal cells to hyperplasia to atypical cells. 2.6% of the women with no NAF (nipple aspiration fluid) developed breast cancer. 4.3% of the women with NAF and normal cells got breast cancer. 5.5% of the women with NAF and epithelial hyperplasia became diagnosed with breast cancer, and 10.3% of women who had NAF and atypical hyperplasia acquired it.

This study is interesting because it takes data from the fluid drawn and compares it to actual results over a period of time. (See Wrensch MR, Petrakis NL, King EB, et al. "Breast cancer incidence in women with abnormal cytology in nipple aspirates of breast fluid." American Journal of Epidemiology 1992; 135: 130-141.)

The follow-up of the women in the study took place for an average of 12.7 years. It would be interesting to know what has happened to these same women over a longer period of time. It is now 2009, thus 29 years since they examined the fluids. I'd also like to know what treatment, if any, these women received after learning the results from their fluids and, also, what type of breast cancer they developed.

If you do a NAF test and have abnormal cells, you should consult with your doctors to see if he/she can know which ductal system has the abnormal cells as well as to discuss further screening and treatment options.

SELF AND CLINICAL EXAMINATIONS

Get to know your breasts. Become comfortable with them. All women should do monthly self breast exams, and it is best to do them at the same time every month, normally a few days after your period. This is when your breasts are least likely to be tender or swollen.

If you no longer have a period, select a day which is easy to remember, like the 1st of each month. It is a good idea to examine your breasts more than once a month, and at different times of the month, to become familiar with how your own breasts feel. If you do this regularly, there is a much better chance for you to notice if anything seems unusual. For more information on how to do a breast self-exam, see www.pph.org and click on Women's Services.

"Clinical breast examinations" are done by a primary care doctor, nurse practitioner, gynecologist, or a surgeon. The surgeon may be your best choice since they examine and then biopsy suspicious areas of the breast. They notice what feels out of the ordinary, and then can confirm whether or not it is problematic with the biopsy they perform. It could be difficult to schedule an appointment with a surgeon, so plan to start out with a primary care doctor, nurse practitioner, or gynecologist who can then refer you to a surgeon if they feel anything unusual.

MAMMOGRAM

A woman's breasts are denser when she is younger because they are preparing to produce milk during her fertile years.

POINTS FROM DR. BARRY:

- **Glands are functional and with age they atrophy due to hormonal changes and disuse.**

After menopause a woman's breasts are generally fattier and less dense. It is easier to see cancer or something suspicious on the mammogram of an older woman as opposed to the denser breast tissue of a younger woman. Thus, mammograms are more effective for older women and older women are at a higher risk for breast cancer merely because they are older.

According to the American Cancer Society Guidelines, women should begin their yearly mammograms at age 40. If you notice anything unusual, then you may need a mammogram more often. It is wise to have a mammogram early, before anything is detected, so you can use it as a baseline of comparison for future mammograms. If anything is out of the ordinary, you have a greater chance of catching it near the beginning.

If you haven't already done so, schedule your baseline mammogram by age 40. Every woman over 40 should have a yearly mammogram and gynecological exam.

To avoid discomfort, it is best to have your mammogram a week or two after your period. You can also ask your technician if they have a special cushioning device called a Mammopad.

Request a digital mammogram rather than a traditional mammogram. It may cost more than a regular one but it appears to be a more effective screening device, with less radiation, than the traditional one.

If you do not have insurance, low cost mammograms are available, contact the American Cancer Society (1-800-227-2345 or www.cancer.org) or the National Breast and Cervical Cancer Early Detection Program (1- 888-842-6355 or www.cdc.gov/cancer/ nbccedp) for more information. Select a month, or a special date each year, to schedule your mammogram so you don't forget to do it.

Women younger than 50 years old are more likely to have a false-negative mammogram than older women. Meaning, they feel something, and or their doctor feels something, but the mammogram doesn't show anything. Until I turned 41 my mammograms never showed anything suspicious, even though I had a palpable/feelable lump or hardness prior to that.

If you are at a high risk of getting breast cancer because of a family history of breast cancer, you are a carrier of the gene mutations BRCA1 or BRCA2 or you have had breast cancer already then you should talk to your doctor about how often you should be getting a mammogram and/or other tests.

If you have a palpable (feelable) lump, then request a mammogram even if you are young. Don't give up if the mammogram does not show anything yet you or your doctor feel something unusual. Err on the side of caution and get it biopsied since this is the only way to know for sure if you have breast cancer.

POINTS FROM DR. BARRY:

- **If you have a palpable lump get it biopsied.**
- **Even the mammogram report will state that palpable lumps should be biopsied even with a negative mammogram.**
- **With a palpable lump the mammogram becomes a screening tool for other suspicious areas.**

Most invasive breast cancer has been growing for six to eight years before it can be detected by a mammogram. (Isn't that comforting.) With that in mind, definitely consider getting a NAF (nipple aspiration fluid) test. (See my discussion of the HALO NAF test.) It can reportedly detect cancerous **cells** six to eight years before cancer is visible on a mammogram.

Again, mammograms do not look at cells. If anything suspicious is found on your mammogram, have it biopsied so the cells can be examined by a pathologist.

It is possible that in the breast cancer's second year it has already begun creating new blood cells to feed the cancer. These new blood vessels can be what allow the cancer to spread. You want to detect cancer as early as possible. Your life is at stake.

POINTS FROM DR. BARRY:

MRI

- **An MRI uses a strong magnet to align electrons within the atoms of the tissue being studied.**
- **Radiowaves are then aimed at the tissue which knocks the electrons out of alignment. The electrons emit energy when they return**

to their alignment and this is measured by
the scanner.
- The result is a picture of the tissues based on
their density and water content.
- It is more useful for soft tissue as
opposed to bone or calcium in contrast to
mammography or a CT scan but it gives a
more detailed picture of the soft tissue than
the other two and does not use ionizing
radiation.
- You still will likely miss any tumors that are
smaller than 1 cm as would be the case with
a CT scan.

POINTS FROM DR. BARRY:

PETscan

- A PETscan is a good tool for screening for
metastases.
- It takes advantage of the fact that cancers
grow more rapidly than most other cells in
the body and as such have a stronger appetite
for glucose-the fuel our cells use to thrive.
- The patient is given a radioactive tainted
analogue of glucose that the cells recognize
as glucose initially but that cannot be fully
utilized as glucose is. (Like putting sugar-
laden gas in your car's gas tank. At first it
will work but quickly it gums up the engine.)
- The Fluorodexoyglucose gets stuck in the
cells and more of it gets stuck in the cancer
cells. It emits radiation that is detected by

a counter and the cancer shows up as "hot spots."
- **A PETscan will sometimes miss lesions in the brain.**

YOUNG WOMEN with a family history of breast cancer, breast or ovarian cancer, or for those with the BRCA1 or BRCA2 gene mutation:

These women should begin monthly self breast exams by 18 years of age and annual or semiannual clinical breast exams by age 25.

They should begin yearly mammograms and/or an MRI between the ages of 25 to 35. The earlier the better, although with younger dense breasts a mammogram may not be too effective. These women need to take special care and find doctors who will create an effective prevention plan for them.

SCREENING STEPS TO TAKE IF YOU NOTICE ANYTHING SUSPICIOUS:

If you feel something odd it may be a lump, so meet with your doctor. You may need to start out with your general practitioner or gynecologist, yet the ideal specialist is a breast surgeon who is more experienced with breast lumps than the others. A surgeon can evaluate your situation more effectively than a nurse practitioner, general family doctor, or even a gynecologist. You will probably need a referral to the surgeon, from one of the other medical providers mentioned.

A doctor may aspirate the area to differentiate between it being a cyst or an actual lump. If it is a cyst it will deflate from the puncture of the needle, and you are likely done unless something else appears out of the ordinary.

Afterward your doctor may request that you have a mammogram and/or an ultrasound. They do not show cells. A radiologist looks for abnormal areas on the mammogram. A biopsy scrutinized by a pathologist or a cytologist under a microscope examines **cells.** (See my section on the HaloNaf test. It also examines cells.)

As a review, an ultrasound is the best choice for younger women who have dense breasts. A mammogram is more effective for older breasts with more fatty tissue as compared to younger, dense breasts. An ultrasound is most effective for observing anything unusual (i.e. a lump) rather than as a diagnostic screening test like a mammogram. Both tests do not look at cells. They provide guidance in examining abnormal areas.

POINTS FROM DR. BARRY:

- **Mammograms have limited usefulness in younger women who generally have dense breasts. It is like looking for a polar bear in a snow storm.**
- **An ultrasound is not a great screening tool. It is better for examining lumps that can be felt and can be used to tell if the lump is solid –a tumor or fluid- a cyst.**

The quality of your mammogram or ultrasound depends on the experience-level of the technician performing your test. Make sure you have your testing done at a place that offers them on a consistent basis with highly-trained technicians

POINTS FROM DR. BARRY:

- **Mammography is the most practical screening tool.**
- **Breasts with implants may impair the radiologist's ability to read the films.**

If you or your doctor notice anything unusual in your breast or something suspicious is viewed on your mammogram, including micro-calcifications, then consider requesting a biopsy to surgically remove the lump or tissue. Then have it analyzed by a pathologist. Do not settle for a needle biopsy. Actually have the lump or suspicious area surgically removed.

I had a needle biopsy and it didn't reveal any abnormalities. I had this procedure just a few months before my breast cancer diagnosis. It can easily miss the actual cancer site and give you a false sense that everything is all right. In the mammogram I had afterward, a few months before my mastectomies, I had so many calcifications that if they had removed them all, my breasts would have looked like Swiss cheese. It just wasn't possible via biopsy to remove all of my calcifications so I chose the mastectomies.

POINTS FROM DR. BARRY:

- **Stereotactic biopsy is an option and is very accurate. Mentally, however, some women prefer to have the lump removed.**

If the biopsy comes back and you find out you have breast cancer, then ask if you have "clean margins." This means the border around the cancer is free of cancer. The bigger the clean margin (area free of cancer), the better. If your report shows a clean margin then depending on the stage of the cancer and other factors, you may or may not need radiation. If you can have partial breast radiation, meaning only to the area that had the cancer, this is optimal. You may also need a sentinel node biopsy (the first lymph nodes that cancer may have spread to are removed and tested for cancer) and/or Tamoxifen or other medications to help prevent a recurrence.

Get the pathologist's report even if you don't have cancer.

POINTS FROM DR. BARRY:

- **A 1 centimeter margin is generally considered adequate, as a clean margin, though there may be instances when this is not possible.**

If the biopsy returns showing you have breast cancer without a clean margin (a roughly 1 centimeter cancer free edge around the cancer), and/or the follow-up mammogram still sees something suspicious then you may need a re-excision (another surgical procedure) to remove more tissue. You may also need to have a sentinel node biopsy.

After the re-excision, if you have a clean margin then you still may need radiation, chemotherapy, or other treatment. If you still do not have a clean margin after the re-excision then you may have to have a mastectomy. Please see my section entitled "Treatment Choices" for more information about the different treatment choices that you may have to choose from if you are at high risk for breast cancer or are diagnosed with breast cancer.

POINTS FROM DR. BARRY:

- **Presently, 4 or more lymph nodes that are positive for cancer means you will need radiation to the axilla. This is currently the standard treatment but it may change with time as new studies are evaluated.**

BIOPSIES

- **A mammogram may see abnormalities but it can't see cells or what actions they are taking.**
- **A surgical biopsy consists of the surgeon removing tissue so a pathologist can later examine the cells in the tissue to see if they are abnormal and to better understand what the cells are doing (i.e. if they are multiplying).**

POINTS FROM DR. BARRY:

- **A histologic study looks at cells under a microscope.**

If something suspicious is detected in a screening test or the surgeon still needs more information afterward (such as a mammogram, ultrasound, MRI or HALO-NAF) then you should have a biopsy. If you have a suspicious lump then GET IT BIOPSIED. Even with our current screening and testing, the best way to know if something is cancerous is to have it removed via a biopsy and then analyzed by a pathologist. Without the biopsy you can not be certain about what is going on in your body.

There are several different types of lumps and most are benign, so don't get freaked out if you find one. Statistically, there are roughly 12 benign lumps for every one cancerous lump in premenopausal women. Unfortunately, in postmenopausal women there is a higher risk for a lump to be cancerous.

If you have breast cancer, you want it diagnosed as early as possible. Do not let a doctor tell you it is nothing and then not follow-up with exams or testing. You must be your own advocate and be persistent. If you feel something is wrong make sure your doctor continues testing until you have definitive answers as in, "No" you don't have breast cancer or "yes" you do have it.

Again, if you notice anything out of the ordinary, the only way to know for sure it is or isn't cancer is to have it biopsied, and not just a needle biopsy. In my situation, I had a needle biopsy and it showed I didn't have breast cancer. My early stage breast cancer, DCIS, wasn't discovered until I had a biopsy which excised my tissue. Then with another biopsy, my doctors found more DCIS.

Since I had been nursing until a few days before my biopsy, I was not given a mammogram. Soon after my biopsies which indicated I had *mutifocal DCIS*, they ordered me a mammogram. My mammogram showed many unusual calcifications. Dr. X wanted the most suspicious areas biopsied, so she sent me for a stereotactic biopsy. I layed face down on a table with my breast sticking through a hole in the table. The technician used my mammogram and other imaging to locate the most suspect areas for analysis. The Radiologist then guided the needle to my numbed breast, inserted it, and pulled out tissue. The procedure felt somewhat uncomfortable and I got a large hematoma in my right breast (softball size mass that didn't go away for months). The results came back benign.

However, after having my breasts removed the pathologist still found about an inch of DCIS which had gone undetected. You must be relentless with your health and your doctors to obtain your answers. IF you have breast cancer, you want it diagnosed right away.

There are several types of biopsies you can have. Please see <u>Dr. Susan Love's Breast Book, 4th edition,</u> starting on page 81 regarding the different types of lumps and which biopsy she recommends.

Dr. Love's book is fairly easy to understand, straightforward, and a wealth of information. If you enjoy learning then read the whole book. If you prefer not to read all 600 plus pages then refer to the table of contents and index; and only read the sections which interest you. As I've mentioned, her book is the "bible" for breast cancer. If you read nothing else, at least review the different types of biopsies and screening tests which are available.

I've written my book to express my feelings and experiences as well as provide you with some basic guidelines to deal with breast cancer, particularly in its early stage. Please do not rely on this book alone. Seek out expert opinions and guidance.

A Brief Overview of BIOPSIES:

- **Needle biopsy: the doctor uses a needle to pull a few cells out of the lump.**
- **There are subcategories of needle biopsies:**
- **a fine needle biopsy is when a doctor uses a fine needle to pull a few cells out of the lump**
- **a larger needle biopsy is when a small portion is cut out of the lump.**

- **Excisional biopsy: the surgeon cuts out the entire lump or suspicious area.**

POINTS FROM DR. BARRY:

- **Other subcategories of biopsies:**
- **Stereotaxis-using x-rays to guide the biopsy to a particular area thus, increasing the accuracy of the biopsy.**
- **Core needle biopsy.**

After your biopsy request and save your pathology report. Even if your lump or suspicious area is removed and benign, keep a copy of your pathology report for future reference. If you had the biopsy after a suspicious finding in your mammogram, then schedule another mammogram a month or two after the biopsy to have a new baseline for future comparison.

I had a needle biopsy in the surgeon's office, and it wasn't a big deal. It showed no cancer. I later had an excisional biopsy in a small surgical room at the doctor's office. She numbed the area, I stayed awake, and we chatted during the procedure. They hooked me up to some monitors, and I felt a bit disgusted by what Dr. X described as she felt inside of my body. While she removed the suspicious area, she noticed something grainy nearby, and that was later discovered to be DCIS. They allowed me to go home a few minutes after the procedure. Overall, this biopsy procedure went smoothly, but I did have some stiffness in my arm for a few days.

The pathologist analyzed my specimen and found the DCIS (early stage non invasive breast cancer.) There was not enough "clean margin" of cancer free tissue around the DCIS, so I had more tissue taken out for analysis via another surgical biopsy.

This time they performed the procedure in a small surgical room and gave me general anesthesia, so I'd sleep through the procedure. Dr. X had to go deeper this time and thus the need to do the procedure in an actual operating room and to put me to sleep. I don't remember the procedure and thankfully woke up soon after they finished. I stayed in recovery for a few hours and then went home. Again, my arm felt stiff, and my motion was restricted for a few days.

DO NOT PUT OFF HAVING A BIOPSY BECAUSE YOU ARE BREASTFEEDING OR PREGNANT. (See my section entitled, "Factors that Contribute to Breast Cancer" where I discuss the increased risks for breast cancer soon after a pregnancy.) It may be messy to operate on a lactating breast, but surgeons should be used to messy and gross things. Read Dr. Barry's point below, to avoid a spontaneous abortion do your best to avoid having general anesthesia. You can have several different types of biopsies without general anesthesia. If you are pregnant and need a biopsy, be sure to clarify this with your doctor.

POINTS FROM DR. BARRY:

- **General anesthesia during pregnancy greatly increases the risk of a spontaneous abortion.**

Keep in mind biopsies may be necessary and are not too painful or intrusive. Nevertheless it is surgery with its potential complications and discomfort. I still think a biopsy which removes tissue is the best way to analyze anything unusual. Always discuss the best course of action with your doctor.

BEFORE YOU AGREE TO HAVE A BIOPSY FIND OUT THE FOLLOWING:

- **Which type of biopsy your surgeon is planning on doing.**
- **Will you require anesthesia. Will you be going to sleep.**
- **Whether or not someone needs to drive you home.**
- **Where your incision will be.**
- **How much tissue they plan on removing.**

- **How big your scar is expected to be.**
- **Will there be any disfigurement (i.e. a large amount of tissue will be removed which may leave one breast significantly smaller than the other).**
- **What to do and not do before and after the procedure.**
- **What to expect in terms of pain and recovery time.**
- **These questions are not meant for vanity reasons. It is important to know what to expect rather than be surprised afterward.**
- **If you are allergic to medications, tape, sutures, or anything else then let your doctors know before your procedure.**

Once again, if your instincts tell you something is wrong; LISTEN. Do not go along with doctors who say everything is fine if they haven't done the proper testing to determine this. A visual exam or even a hands-on physical exam of the breasts is not enough. A biopsy is the only sure way to know if something suspicious on a mammogram is cancer or not. You must be your own advocate. Unfortunately, some doctors fail to diagnose or even misdiagnose illnesses. You must be persistent and get a second opinion if you need to.

POINTS FROM DR. BARRY:

- **A biopsy is only practical:**
- **In the presence of a palpable (feelable) mass or nipple discharge.**
- **In the presence of a radiographic abnormality.**

D. TREATMENT CHOICES

When deciding which treatment is right for you, gather as much helpful information as possible. Try not to overanalyze everything. Make the best decision for **yourself,** not for your doctor or significant other. Really think about the risks you can live with, what procedure gives you the best chance of survival and the least chance of recurrence, while weighing the possible side effects for each option. Do not choose the procedure which seems easiest.

There are several treatments for breast cancer. You may only need one, or you might require a combination of several treatments. I will give you a brief overview of the main Western medicine treatments for breast cancer. Please feel free to do more reading and research on each treatment that may pertain to you.

In brief, if you get breast cancer or are at a high risk of getting breast cancer and are trying to avoid getting it then you will probably select from the following treatments:

D. TYPES OF BREAST CANCER TREAMENT

1. SURGICAL TREATMENTS
- **Lumpectomy/Breast Sparing**
- **Wide Excision**
- **Mastectomy**
  - **Simple**
  - **Total**
  - **Modified radical (rarely radical)**
- **Sentinel Node Biopsy - a diagnostic test to check for cancer in your lymph nodes. It is a surgical procedure which can be performed on its own or during the surgical procedures above.**
- **Reconstruction - Not a treatment yet can be done following the above surgical procedures.**
  - **Most Common Types of Reconstruction**

1. Implants-Expanders and then implants
2. TRAM FLAP
3. Dorsal Flap-Latissimus Dorsi flap with expander or implant

2. SYSTEMIC THERAPY

- **Chemotherapy**
- **Hormone Therapy**
  - ○ **Tamoxifen**
  - ○ **Aromatase Inhibitors**
- **Targeted Therapies**

3. RADIATION

4. COMPLIMENTARY BUT NOT ALTERNATIVE TREATMENTS

I will primarily discuss treatment choices related to DCI since this was my diagnosis, and I focused the majority of my research on this condition. Even if you have another breast cancer you can benefit from my research and discussions because the treatment for most breast cancers involve similar options.

SURGICAL TREATMENTS

According to the National Cancer Institute website http://www.
cancer.gov/cancertopics/breast-cancer-surgery-choices most women
who have DCIS or Stage I, IIA, IIB, or IIIA breast cancer have **three**
basic SURGERY choices.

- **Breast sparing surgery (lumpectomy, wide excision)**
- **Mastectomy**
- **Mastectomy with breast reconstruction surgery**

These choices for treating early stage breast cancer shocked me.
I kept hoping more research would lead me to a better treatment
choice. Sadly I didn't find one.

LUMPECTOMY/ BREAST SPARING

Breast-sparing surgery means the surgeon removes your cancer
and some normal tissue around it. They need a cancer-free margin (a
specific area around the cancer which is cancer free). The main goal
is to rid the cancer, but your breast should look much like it did before
the surgery. Some other words used for breast-sparing surgery are
"lumpectomy", "partial mastectomy", "quadrantectomy" or "breast-
conserving surgery."

After breast-sparing surgery, many women also need radiation
therapy, chemotherapy and/or hormone therapy such as Tamoxifen
or an Aromatose inhibitor. (Do not confuse these hormone therapies
with hormone replacement therapy, controversial methods used for
postmenopausal symptoms.) The goal is to prevent a recurrence of
cancer in the same breast.

POINTS FROM DR. BARRY:

- **Those with invasive breast cancer who opt for a lumpectomy must, by protocol, get breast radiation.**

WIDE EXCISION

Another treatment choice for DCIS is wide excision, which is the removal of the entire area with DCIS and a clean margin (a cancer free area of tissue around the DCIS). The amount of breast tissue removed will be determined by looking at your mammogram, ultrasound, and previous biopsies.

With DCIS there isn't a lump, so it is not a lumpectomy. In my case I had a thickening which kept coming back and the DCIS was right next to it.

In us smaller breasted women, a wide excision might be similar to having a mastectomy. My doctors never mentioned this treatment choice. Check with your doctor to see how much of your breast will exist after this procedure, if this is your treatment option. Also, ask about any scarring you might experience, and if you will need any breast reconstruction after the wide excision.

POINTS FROM DR. BARRY:

- **Also ask what changes to expect after radiating the breast post lumpectomy.**

MASTECTOMY

Since you're this far along in my book, I assume you have read the more detailed description of my breast cancer. Just in case you skimmed through, I will give you a brief overview. While nursing my son I noticed something hard on the right side of the armpit area of my right breast. I was told that I couldn't get a mammogram since I was still nursing. I had an ultrasound which showed nothing suspicious; a needle biopsy which didn't reveal any cancer; and visited an acupuncturist who assured me I didn't have breast cancer. I still decided to have a biopsy and through this procedure the doctors found DCIS, early stage, non-invasive breast cancer.

POINTS FROM DR. BARRY:

- **I do not believe that an acupuncturist has a way to find cancer.**

Without a clean margin, the surgeon needed to perform a re-excision. They then found more DCIS with a clean margin. I then had a mammogram which showed extensive calcifications in both breasts. The most suspicious calcifications were removed by stereotactic biopsies, and these biopsies indicated no cancer. After much research and deliberation, I chose a bilateral mastectomy (having both breasts removed) since I felt this would give me the best chance of survival with the least chance of a recurrence. After my ongoing research, I am still happy with my decision.

In a mastectomy the surgeon removes as much of your breast tissue as possible and most likely will remove your nipple and areola (the circle around your nipple). It is possible to have a mastectomy and keep your nipples. However, you then run a risk of getting cancer in them. Since the surgeon cannot remove every breast cell, you could get still get breast cancer even after a double mastectomy. .

After a mastectomy you may need radiation therapy, chemotherapy, hormone therapy, or all three types of therapy. Thankfully, because they found no invasive cancer in my removed breasts or lymph nodes, I didn't need any of these additional treatments.

There are different types of mastectomies:

- **Total mastectomy/skin sparing mastectomy: The surgeon removes as much breast tissue as possible and may take out some lymph nodes under your arm. The muscle and as much skin as possible is left. I had this done, and they also removed the sentinel lymph node (the main lymph node most likely to have cancer) from each armpit area.**

- Modified radical mastectomy: The surgeon removes as much of your breast tissue as possible, many of the lymph nodes under your arm, the lining over your chest muscles, and, if needed, a small amount of chest muscle.
- Double or Bilateral Mastectomy: The surgeon removes both of your breasts. I chose this even though I had only been diagnosed with early stage breast cancer in my right breast.

Things you should know:

- Even after a mastectomy cancer can come back in the scar area or the chest wall.
- Your surgeon will remove as much breast tissue as possible, but they can't remove all tissue and all cells.
- Many doctors do not favor mastectomy and think it should be done in very limited circumstances. I disagree as I explained earlier regarding why I chose a mastectomy over radiation followed by Tamoxifen.
- You will need to make the decision which is right for you.
- After your mastectomy move your arm and do easy exercises as soon as your doctor allows you to do so, the sooner the better.
- Talk to your doctor about what you should and should not do.
- Getting your movement back and relieving the stiffness will help you recover, but do not overdo it.

SENTINEL NODE BIOPSY

According to the National Cancer Institutes' website, a sentinel lymph node biopsy is the "Removal and examination of the sentinel node(s) (the first lymph node(s) to which cancer cells are likely to spread from a primary tumor. To identify the sentinel lymph node(s), the surgeon injects a radioactive substance, blue dye, or both near the tumor. The surgeon then uses a scanner to find the sentinel lymph node(s) containing the radioactive substance or looks for the lymph node(s) stained with dye. The surgeon then removes the sentinel node(s) to check for the presence of cancer cells."

- **A sentinel node biopsy may be used in conjunction with a mastectomy, or may be used with a lumpectomy, wide excision, or radiation.**
- **The sentinel node biopsy involves taking one to three lymph nodes, the ones more likely to have breast cancer.**
- **A full axillary node dissection involves the removal of 15-20 lymph nodes from under the armpit.**
- **Due to less lymph nodes being taken out in the sentinel node biopsy, as compared to a full axillary node dissection, recovery should be much easier and there should be less complications.**
- **Radioactive dye is injected into your breast area about two hours before your surgery. The blue dye then travels from the tumor to the lymph node. Make your doctor aware if you have an allergy to sulfa, or you may suffer a bad reaction to the dye.**

POINTS FROM DR. BARRY:

- **A sentinel node biopsy is an alternative to a lymph node dissection.**
- **It is used when lymph nodes are not yet known to already have cancer.**

Your surgeon must be skilled to perform this relatively new surgery. Don't be afraid to ask your surgeon about their experience doing sentinel node biopsies. You want a surgeon who has completed more than 20 procedures with a success rate of finding the sentinel node at least 85% of the time. For example, if they have done 20 procedures, they should have been successful at least 17 times. If your surgeon doesn't meet this criteria, then seriously consider a different surgeon.

If possible, it is better to get a sentinel node biopsy than a full axillary node dissection because you will most likely have fewer side effects. You will less likely have problems with movement, or with feeling in your arm and shoulder. You're also least likely to have lymphedema (something you definitely want to avoid) with the sentinel node biopsy.

If your lymph nodes come back positive for cancer after having the sentinel node biopsy then you may need an axillary node dissection, but only if it is necessary. Do not choose this because you have a surgeon unskilled in performing a sentinel node biopsy. Find one who is.

If you previously had chemotherapy, radiation, or a lot of breast surgery, you may not be able to get a sentinel node biopsy. My surgeon told me that she wasn't sure if she could perform a sentinel node biopsy on my right side due to my many previous biopsies. Fortunately she found a way to perform the procedure and took out the sentinel node and one other lymph node from my right side as well as the sentinel node from my left side. Thankfully, they came back cancer free, so I did not need more lymph nodes removed or any additional treatments other than the bilateral mastectomies.

To check on a clinical trial regarding sentinel node dissection with or without full axillary dissection (removing more than the sentinel lymph node) see www.clinicaltrials.gov There are many trials listed and some are seeking new participants.

RECONSTRUCTION

If you have a mastectomy, in most cases you will be able to have breast reconstruction surgery if you choose to. According to Federal law, if you have a mastectomy then your insurance must pay for reconstruction if you want it. They may have restrictions on when you can have it done as well as the type of reconstruction you can request. Fully investigate this before you make your decision to have a mastectomy. Check with your insurance company and doctors before making your treatment decision.

POINTS FROM DR. BARRY:

- **It is the doctor and patient who make the reconstruction issues.**
- **It is not a restriction imposed by the insurance company.**

The reconstruction portion of the surgery is done by a reconstructive plastic surgeon who will give you a new breast-like shape. A few months later your reconstructive surgeon can create a nipple from your tissue and then add a tattoo that looks like the areola (the dark area around your nipple). They look fake up close, but I am fine with that.

If you do not have implants but have the skin, tissue and muscle taken from another area of your body, you might be able to get softer, bigger breasts than when implants are used. This does involve more extensive surgeries to the breast area and also to the area where the skin, muscle, and tissue are taken from, ie. butt, back, thighs, or abdomen.

In an article entitled "Breast Cancer: Know the Surgery Options-Study Shows Many Patients Aren't Told About Reconstruction." By Salynn Boyles and Reviewed by Louise Chang, M.D. found at www.webmd.com/breast-cancer/news/20071221/breast-cancer-know-the-surgery-options?ecd=wnl_brc_010808 they indicate that researchers surveyed almost 1,200 early stage breast cancer patients eligible for breast conserving lumpectomy or mastectomy around the year 2002. Only 33% of the women said that they discussed breast reconstruction with their general surgeon during their initial decision making meeting. Patients who discussed reconstruction with their surgeon were four times more likely to have a mastectomy than a lumpectomy.

According to plastic surgeon, Amy Alderman, MD, who led the study team, women must be fully informed of their surgical choices before they decide on a treatment course. She mentions there are pros and cons for each treatment choice, and the doctors need to share this information with their patients.

TYPES OF RECONSTRUCTION

IMPLANTS

The tissue expansion method of reconstruction puts an expander, implant, filled with saline (salt water) or silicone gel under your skin or chest muscle to build a new breast-like shape, mound. A tissue expander is placed in during or after the mastectomy. Reconstruction surgery may take one and a half to two hours in addition to the time for the mastectomy.

If you have this type of reconstruction, if possible, I recommend your expanders be placed in at the same time as your mastectomy. Personally, I did not want to leave the table without any breasts. This also avoids another surgery to put in temporary implants.

I also suggest you **NOT have a mastectomy as an outpatient**. I could not have gone home right after surgery. I felt weak, and they had me attached to an IV, a catheter and drains. I recommend you stay in the hospital with professionals looking after you decreasing your risk for complications and infections.

According to the movie I watched at my reconstructive surgeon's office, the expanders don't normally limit any movement. I disagree. At first you may experience pain doing some very common things, like cutting a bagel or shutting a window. Thus, you may limit your movements due to this discomfort. The pain may not only arise from the implants. It can result from a combination of the mastectomies and the reconstruction. I found it impossible to know where the discomfort originated since the two surgeries were done at basically the same time.

The temporary implants are gradually filled with more saline every two or three weeks. They have ports and the reconstructive surgeon injects them with saline and the implant expands. If it ruptures, you'll most likely realize it. At some point later the temporary implants, breast expanders, are surgically removed and replaced with permanent implants. Then nipples are constructed. The implant can go behind your muscle. The skin is used from your own breast area so your size can be limited by how much skin is available after your mastectomy.

Some women may have little or no feeling in their breast area after a mastectomy because their nerves have been cut during surgery. About a year after my mastectomies most of the feeling returned to my breast area. There are still a few areas of my breast that do not have sensation. There are some tiny hairs and spots on my breast I had been annoyed with in the past. Now I am glad to see them as it makes the new breast mounds seem more like my breasts. It is comforting to see my own skin.

Your skin might feel numb when it is touched after a mastectomy. If I am feeling around my breast area, I sense it. If someone else touches me, for the most part, I am aware of it. Ask your partner not to touch you too firmly because may hurt you.

My daughter and I sometimes played a game to see if I could feel her touching my breast. I'd close my eyes, and she may or may not have been touching me. I had to tell her when I thought I had been touched. Most of the time I could distinguish her touch but certain areas of my new breasts did not have much, if any sensation. Some areas may actually feel painful. Over time you can have some or most of the feeling restored to your breast area.

Breast implants may not last forever, and you may need more surgery later on to replace them. Implants can cause problems such as breast hardness, breast pain, and infection. The implant may also break, move, or shift. You may also get a ridged look to your breast area. These problems can occur soon after surgery or years later. I like to think positively and assume my implants will be fine for a long time. My implants haven't caused me any inconvenience.

The movie I watched at Dr. S's office mentioned there is less surgical risk with implants as compared to other kinds of reconstruction. With implants one has a smaller incision so the healing and recuperation is expected to be more rapid.

TRAM FLAP

Another way of doing breast reconstruction is the TRAM flap reconstruction method which uses your natural tissue from your own stomach. This tissue is used to build a breast and according to the movie at the reconstructive surgeon's office, it requires four to six hours of surgery (in addition to the time for the mastectomy), three to seven days in the hospital and four to six weeks of recovery. An incision is made into your lower abdomen, and your stomach muscles are tunneled up to your chest. Skin is also taken from your stomach area. If you are too thin, too obese, smoke, or have other serious health problems, this method of reconstruction may not be an option for you.

There are some downsides to the TRAM flap method of reconstruction. The newly created flap may not survive; you can have abdominal problems with the scar; your belly button could die because of an inadequate blood supply; you could have a hernia; and the flap might be lumpy. Because muscle is taken from your stomach to build a new breast mound, the surgery may decrease the strength in your remaining stomach muscles. This is major surgery and will most likely take you longer to heal than if you have the breast implant method. As in any surgery, you may get an infection or have difficulty healing in the surgical areas.

The benefits of this type of reconstruction are you avoid the risks of implants by using your own natural tissue, and your breasts may feel softer than with implants. You also may get a bit of a tummy tuck, and your new breast may last the rest of your life without the need of additional surgery to replace implants.

LATTISSIMUS DORSI FLAP

There is also another method called the lattissimus dorsi flap/back flap where they take tissue and skin from your back and create a breast with it. This is also more extensive surgery than having implants inserted.

Whatever the method of reconstruction, a nipple can later be created with your own tissue, and tattoos can be used to create the appearance of an areola. You can read about my experience with both of these in the beginning section of this book. Remember, you don't have to get new nipples and/or areolas if you don't want more procedures.

SIDE EFFECTS FROM SURGERY

- **You may get a frozen shoulder, especially if you have had a full axillary lymph node dissection, the removal of the lymph nodes under your armpit.**
- **Talk to your doctor about what exercises you can begin after your surgery. The sooner you can start, the better it will be for your arms and shoulder in terms of stiffness and getting your full range of motion back. Just make sure you don't overdo it.**

- You may need to have physical therapy if you have problems with your arms or shoulders. You may also want to try massage and acupuncture.
- Of course, you will have scarring after surgery. It will most likely not be as bad as you expect it to be. Mine isn't.
- You may also get lymphedema (swelling of the hand or arm).

LYMPHEDEMA

- You may get lymphedema from the removal of your lymph nodes, from radiation, infections, or surgeries.
- The lymphedema can be swelling in your fingers (which I have had for over three years) and/or swelling in your arms.
- It may be a permanent or temporary condition. It can happen soon after surgery or a few years later.
- It may be very minor or it can be more severe swelling.
- Exercise caution to avoid this problem.

According to **Dr. Love's Breast Book**, 4th edition, recent studies have shown if you have a sentinel node biopsy (the head lymph node that cancer may have spread to is removed to biopsy it for cancer) you have a 2-6% chance of getting lymphedema which is considerably lower than the 17-34% chance of acquiring lymphedema if the full axillary dissection is done. Thus, you are less likely to have lymphedema after a sentinel node biopsy where they only take out one to a few lymph nodes as compared to the full axillary lymph node dissection where 15-20 lymph nodes from under your armpit may be removed. Although unlikely, it is still possible to get lymphedema with a sentinel node biopsy.

AVOIDING LYMPHEDEMA

- Garden with gloves on to avoid cuts.
- Do not reach into a hot oven.
- Avoid all cuts to the hands, fingers, and arms. If you cut yourself use an antibiotic ointment right away to avoid infections. If you get an infection then see your doctor.

POINTS FROM DR. BARRY:

- I think that most doctors would agree that in the absence of an infection, oral or IV antibiotics are overkill and likely to breed resistant organisms.
- It may be enough to just wash and dress the area regularly and use an antibiotic ointment.
- If the area gets infected then see your doctor right away.

- I avoid manicures. Having them is up to you and your doctor.
- Avoid trauma to the side which had a mastectomy. Have blood draws, injections, and blood pressure on the unaffected side. If you had a bilateral mastectomy then have blood drawn from your feet, injections in your buttocks, and blood pressure on your calf. Check with your doctor for other locations.
- Try not to carry heavy objects on that side, especially with your arm down as when carrying grocery bags.
- Carry a light purse.
- Try not to gain weight after surgery.
- If you do experience swelling, elevate your arm.

- **See your doctor with any symptoms since it is best to catch this early.**
- **Talk to your doctor about physical therapy, exercise, massage, and wearing a compression bandage, glove, on your hands and arms, especially on airplanes.**

SURGERY SCHEDULING

If at all possible, schedule any surgery during the second half of your menstrual cycle. It is possible that new blood vessels grow faster in the first half of your cycle. Thus, you may bleed less, and the cancer could have less opportunity to spread during a surgery arranged later in your cycle. Anything you can do to improve your situation is worth it especially when all it involves is planning.

POINTS FROM DR. BARRY:

- **I find this an interesting idea.**

SYSTEMIC THERAPY

- **Systemic therapy is something that treats you by circulating through your whole body.**
- **It doesn't just circulate through a specific area such as the breast.**
- **Chemotherapy, hormone therapy and targeted therapies are all types of systemic therapies.**

CHEMOTHERAPY

The goal of chemotherapy is to kill cancer cells and to decrease the risk of a recurrence of breast cancer. Do your research and ask a lot of questions. There is a lot to know about chemotherapy including the potential side effects and benefits from receiving it.

In chemotherapy, chemicals are given to treat the cancer by preventing the cells from dividing. Chemotherapy kills cells yet, unfortunately, it does not just destroy cancer cells, it also eliminates hair and bone marrow cells. This is likely why people often lose their hair while on it. I know several people who recently had chemotherapy for bladder and breast cancer. They didn't lose their hair, so maybe the process is being refined to only kill the cancer cells rather than the good cells.

POINTS FROM DR. BARRY:

- **Cancer cells divide rapidly as do hair, nail and blood cells and cells that line the intestines. Hence, the side effects of hair falling out, low blood count and diarrhea may be possible when getting chemotherapy.**

The goal of chemotherapy is to substantially reduce the number of cancer cells so your immune system can manage the cancer cells which remain.

You may need to consider chemotherapy if your breast cancer has spread into your lymph nodes or other parts of your body.

Some additional points about chemotherapy you should know:

- **Chemotherapy might accelerate menopause. The closer you are to being in menopause, the more likely you will go into menopause.**
- **Chemotherapy may work best on women who are premenopausal since it often puts them into at least a temporary menopause which affects their hormones in a positive way with regard to breast cancer.**
- **Remember, the less menstrual cycles we have the better for reducing the risk of breast cancer.**
- **If your period does not return, then you will be infertile.**

- **Besides the effects of the chemotherapy on the cancer, not getting a period may help reduce the risk of a recurrence or the spreading of breast cancer by reducing your estrogen production.**
- **Even if a woman's period comes back after chemotherapy, she may have fertility issues.**

If chemotherapy is a treatment choice for you thoroughly research what to expect, along with the side effects you may have, BEFORE you start chemotherapy. There are different types of chemotherapy so find out what you will be taking and make an informed decision.

HORMONE THERAPY

As I've mentioned before, I believe controlling **estrogen** is the key to preventing and/or managing breast cancer.

POINTS FROM DR. BARRY:

- **Well, sort of. Once you have breast cancer, if it is a bad one, even a total shut down of estrogen might not control it.**

- Do not confuse hormone therapy with HRT (hormone **REPLACEMENT** therapy). HRT is used for menopausal symptoms and may cause breast cancer in some women. (See my discussion of HRT in the section entitled, "Factors that May Contribute to Breast Cancer.")
- Hormone therapy is the giving of hormones, or the manipulation of your own hormones to decrease the growth of tissue or tumor sensitive to those particular hormones.
- The goal is to deprive the tumor/tissue of estrogen so the cancer can't grow and may even die without this food source.

- Hormone Therapy may have less side-effects than chemotherapy and can be easier to take since it is available in pill form.

POINTS FROM DR. BARRY:

- **Hormone therapy is sometimes appropriate as a first line agent - particularly in Stage 0 or Stage I breast cancer.**
- **It is usually used as adjunct therapy in Stage III or Stage IV breast cancer.**

In hormone therapy, hormones or drugs which affect your hormones are given to try and prevent or delay a recurrence and prevent metastasizing, the spreading of the cancer to organs other than the breast. Hormone therapy may be able to control or even destroy cancer cells.

In my opinion, your lump or tissue MUST BE TESTED to discover if it is positive for receptors to the hormones estrogen and progesterone. If your tumor/tissue is not sensitive to these hormones, then blocking them probably won't be helpful at all. Why chance the potential side effects for little to no benefit from taking the hormones? If your lump, tissue, IS sensitive to hormones, then this treatment may be beneficial for you.

Be sure you understand the above paragraph and discuss this with your doctor. Find out if you are hormone-receptor-positive or negative. Muster up your courage to ask questions. You must ensure you have treatment designed with YOU in mind, given your particular needs and circumstances.

POINTS FROM DR. BARRY:

- **Hormone receptor tests detect all surface receptors for estrogen and progesterone as well as Her 2 neu.**

- Estrogen binds to the end of the receptor and causes cell division.
- Tamoxifen blocks estrogen from binding to the receptor.
- We don't have any clinically useful progesterone blockers.
- It is not clear what the relationship of progesterone is to breast cancer.
- The drug Herceptin blocks the Her receptor.
- A woman's receptor status is useful in determining her prognosis.
- It is simplistic to say that estrogen is the villain in causing breast cancer. If we aggressively eliminated estrogen from all women there would be no procreation and the species would cease to exist. Also, if we eliminate estrogen from women's bodies, severe osteoporosis rates would probably soar.
- It is clear that certain types of HRT are risky and need to be avoided or at least not entered into lightly. Consider red wine- a little bit seems to reduce heart disease but a lot leads to alcoholism, cirrhosis and premature death.

TAMOXIFEN

- One type of hormone therapy DECREASES the production of estrogen, and the other hormone therapy BLOCKS the estrogen receptor on the cell.
- Tamoxifen is reportedly the best known drug for BLOCKING estrogen which attempts to enter

the breast, and it may also prevent estrogen from reaching cancer cells which have metastasized (spread).

- However, while stopping the estrogen from entering the breast, Tamoxifen may act like estrogen in other organs such as the uterus and the bones.
- Taking Tamoxifen may increase the risk of uterine cancer, blood clots as well as cause hot flashes and other side effects.

POINTS FROM DR. BARRY:

- Tamoxifen belongs to a class of drugs called SERM's-selective estrogen receptor modulators.
- Tamoxifen "modulates" the estrogen receptor. Sometimes that would be to bind to the receptor and block it from stimulation by estrogen as in breast cancer. Sometimes that is to bind to the receptor and stimulate the receptor as in bone and uterus.
- Tamoxifen apparently blocks estrogen in breast tissue but acts like estrogen in bone and uterus. In bone, it inhibits osteoclasts, cells that break down bone and contribute to bone loss. In the uterus it stimulates the endometrium like estrogen and increases the risk of endometrial cancer.
- Tamoxifen should block all estrogen receptors, breast or otherwise.
- Hot flashes with menopause are from lower estrogen levels.

You may help prevent breast cancer, or a recurrence, by taking Tamoxifen or other drugs and/or treatments, but you then may acquire another illness or ailment due to the treatment. Thoroughly evaluate the potential benefits versus the risks for each treatment choice.

You can only take Tamoxifen for up to five years and the longer you take it, the more extended protection you will have in avoiding breast cancer. The benefits continue even after you stop taking the Tamoxifen. It has been studied more than similar drugs. If you experience negative side effects with Tamoxifen, then talk to your doctor about your other drug choices. Also, find out from your doctor if you are estrogen-receptor-positive thus, sensitive to the hormone, estrogen.

Please keep in mind Tamoxifen may be of little or no benefit if your tumor, tissue, is estrogen-receptor-negative. If your tumor, tissue, is not sensitive to estrogen then it is not likely to help you by blocking estrogen from the area. Thus, if you are estrogen-receptor-negative, you probably DO NOT want to take Tamoxifen since it appears not to benefit you. If you are estrogen-receptor-negative, estrogen doesn't seem to be what is causing your tumor to grow. Estrogen nourishes only certain cancer cells to grow, those which are sensitive to estrogen.

If your tumor, tissue, is estrogen-receptor-positive then Tamoxifen may benefit you whether you are pre-menopausal or post-menopausal. It also may help you whether you have cancer in your lymph nodes or not. Studies have proven that women who take Tamoxifen have less recurrences and fewer cancers in the opposite breast.

YOU MUST TALK TO YOUR DOCTOR about Tamoxifen and the prior discussion, and do not take potentially harmful drugs without knowing if they will actually benefit you.

I wasn't told if my DCIS tissue was estrogen-receptor-positive or negative to help me make my treatment choice. I will give my oncologist the benefit of the doubt that he knew Tamoxifen should only have been offered to me if my tissue had been tested, and it came back estrogen-receptor-positive. However, I learned this information AFTER making my treatment choice and having my bilateral mastectomies. I want YOU to know this information and ask questions BEFORE you make your treatment choice.

POSSIBLE SIDE EFFECTS OF TAMOXIFEN

Some of the possible side effects of taking Tamoxifen are:

- **An increased risk of getting uterine cancer.**
- **One of the most serious side effects, uterine cancer, is more common in women over 50.**
- **Tamoxifen blocks estrogen from entering the breasts but may act like estrogen in the uterus. Tamoxifen can increase the risk for uterine cancer**
- **An increased risk for strokes.**
- **An increased risk for heart attacks.**
- **An increased risk of phlebitis.**
- **An increased risk of pulmonary embolus which I believe means a blood clot in the main pulmonary artery.**
- **Hot flashes - About 50% of the women who take Tamoxifen have them.**
- **Fluid retention**
- **Vaginal discharge**
- **For pre-menopausal women Tamoxifen increases the risk of gynecological problems, and they shouldn't get pregnant while taking Tamoxifen because it can hurt the fetus.**

There are many potential side effects, so only women with a fairly high risk for breast cancer should consider this treatment. If you begin Tamoxifen, or any other drug or treatment, and you encounter side effects, definitely discuss other options with your doctor.

It is most important to realize you can decrease the risk for breast cancer but may increase the risk for uterine cancer and other illnesses by taking Tamoxifen. Discuss your individual benefits and risks of taking Tamoxifen and other treatments with your doctor. If you cure your breast cancer with Tamoxifen, it may make sense to take it. But to take it as a preventive measure for the possibility of getting breast cancer may not make sense. By taking Tamoxifen you could acquire something worse than the breast cancer you want to prevent. The higher your probability for breast cancer, then the more it is worth risking the possible side effects of Tamoxifen.

AROMATASE INHIBITORS FOR POSTMENOPAUSAL WOMEN

- **Aromatase Inhibitors are another type of hormone therapy.**
- **Aromatase Inhibitors are taken in a pill form, like Tamoxifen.**
- **Aromatase Inhibitors are more common, yet they are relatively new. Since they have only been taken for about the last ten years, all of the benefits and side effects are still unknown.**
- **Aromatase Inhibitors do not block estrogen production by the ovaries, but they can block other tissues from making estrogen.**

According to the National Cancer Institute website http://www. cancer.gov/cancertopics/aromatase-inhibitors , "Many breast tumors are 'estrogen sensitive', meaning the hormone estrogen helps them to grow. Aromatase Inhibitors can help block the growth of these tumors by lowering the amount of estrogen in the body. Estrogen is produced by the ovaries and other tissues of the body, using a substance called aromatase."

If estrogen is produced by the ovaries, it follows that removing your ovaries could decrease your risk for breast cancer. (See my discussion of this under Gene testing.) Again, our ovaries are a main source of our estrogen production.

Furthermore, the article states that Aromatase Inhibitors are primarily used in women whose ovaries no longer produce estrogen due to MENOPAUSE.

Three Aromatase Inhibitors are currently approved by the U. S. Food and Drug Administration. They are Anastrazole (Arimidex), Exemestane (Aromasin) and Letrozole (Femara). The Aromatase Inhibitors Anastrozole (Arimidex) and Letrozole (Femara) BLOCK the aromatase enzyme on a reversible basis versus Exemestane (Aromasin) which permanently INACTIVATES the aromatase enzyme.

Tamoxifen (Nolvadex) works differently than aromatase inhibitiors. Tamoxifen **BLOCKS** the estrogen which allows an estrogen-sensitive tumor to grow. Aromatase Inhibitors DECREASE the amount of estrogen being **PRODUCED** by the body, not the ovaries.

I printed out an article on Aromatase Inhibitors from the internet on May 24, 2006, a few weeks after my breast cancer diagnosis. When I read the above information on Aromatase Inhibitors in October of 2007, it didn't seem familiar. All of this breast cancer material can be so overwhelming.

The article is entitled, "Breakthroughs in Breast Cancer Treatments- New Findings are Showing Progress in Hormonal and Targeted Breast Cancer Therapies." By Emma Hitt, PhD and reviewed by Cynthia Haines, MD. Please see www.webmd.com/content/pages/24/113001.htm

It discusses advances in hormonal therapy for postmenopausal women. According to the article, Tamoxifen has been used to treat early-stage breast cancer since the 1980's. Recently, a new class of drugs called Aromatase Inhibitors have been proven to produce better results when compared directly with Tamoxifen. "Aromatase Inhibitors, indicated for use in POSTMENOPAUSAL women, act by blocking the formation of estrogen, which fuels the growth of "hormone receptor-positive" breast cancers."

The article discusses different Aromatase Inhibitors studies. In one study patients took Tamoxifen and then later took Femara, a placebo. The results suggest there is a risk of recurrence after completing a five-year course of Tamoxifen, but benefit can be gained from taking Femara, even when there is a delay between its initiation and the conclusion of taking Tamoxifen.

According to the article, "Positive results have also been demonstrated with Arimidex, another aromatase inhibitor, in the treatment of early-stage breast cancer. One study found that switching to Arimidex after two to three years of Tamoxifen was linked to better survival without disease recurrence after five years compared with staying on Tamoxifen for five years." According to this article, "similar findings have been reported for Aromasin."

Discuss Aromatase Inhibitors with your doctor and visit the websites I have provided for more research and articles about Aromatase Inhibitors. Another site you may want to go to is: http://www.cancer.gov/cancertopics/treatment/breast/aromatase-inhibitors0307

Aromatase Inhibitors are relatively new drugs, yet thus far they have reported positive results in studies on POSTMENOPAUSAL WOMEN WITH ESTROGEN POSITIVE metastatic disease and other POSTMENOPAUSAL WOMEN WITH ESTROGEN POSITIVE breast cancer. Note: all of these women had tissue, lumps, which were ESTROGEN-RECEPTOR-POSITIVE, meaning they were sensitive to estrogen.

Since Tamoxifen can only be taken for five years, postmenopausal women might want to try one of these Aromatase Inhibitors after they finish Tamoxifen, especially if they are at a high risk of recurrence.

Studies are also underway to discover if POSTMENOPAUSAL women can benefit as much by taking an Aromatase Inhibitor alone, without first taking Tamoxifen. Thus, for POSTMENOPAUSAL WOMEN WHO ARE ESTROGEN-RECEPTOR-POSITIVE, their first choice may be an Aromatose Inhibitor without Tamoxifen.

Many distinctions need to be taken into account for each type of breast cancer. Also, each woman has her own needs and circumstances, so ensure you talk to your doctor about which treatment is optimal for you. Obtaining a second opinion from another doctor is also encouraged. I think with whichever treatment choice you ultimately select, your mind plays one of the most pivotal roles in your healing process. If you trust your doctors and believe in the treatment you receive, you will have a much higher success rate than if you harbor any doubts about your medical treatment. The mind and the human body work together as a team and are amazing.

ZOLADEX/LUPRON/GOSERELIN

Goserelin, Zoladex, and Lupron are basically the same drug/hormone therapy but are delivered to the patient in different ways. Zoladex is a pellet that is injected monthly under the skin of the abdomen and is said to block the pituitary gland from producing hormones which stimulate the ovary; sending women into a reversible menopause. Lupron is injected every one to three months and Goserelin is a nasal spray.

The less menstrual cycles a woman has, the fewer estrogen fluctuations she will experience. This would have a positive effect on lumps or breast tissue sensitive to estrogen and other hormones. Side effects of these drugs may include hot flashes, weight gain, and other menopausal symptoms

TARGETED THERAPIES

- **An important breakthrough in cancer treatment has been the introduction of so-called "targeted" therapies.**
- **Targeted therapies are designed to hone in on the cancer cells while leaving the healthy cells untouched.**
- **Targeted Therapies are antibodies, drugs, used to block specific enzymes or proteins in order to reduce the malignant potential of the cancer cell.**

203

- **An example of a targeted therapy is Herceptin (Trastuzumab).**

The article entitled, "Breakthroughs in Breast Cancer Treatments - New findings are showing progress in hormonal and targeted breast cancer therapies," by Emma Hitt, PhD and reviewed by Cynthia Haines, MD discusses "targeted therapies." Please see

www.webmd.com/content/pages/24/113001.htm

The above article states, "Herceptin, an effective targeted therapy for breast cancer, attaches to a protein on the surface of breast cancer cells called HER2 that transmits growth-stimulating signals to cells. By blocking the actions of HER2, Herceptin slows or stops the growth of tumor cells. Herceptin is effective in tumors that express large amounts of the HER2 protein (described as HER2-positive), which is the case in about 25% of patients."

Thus, it might make sense to take Herceptin if your tumor or tissue has large amounts of the HER2 protein.

The article continues to discuss some clinical trials using Herceptin in early stage breast cancer and when used with or without chemotherapy.

Herceptin can increase the risk of heart problems. Please see the article for more information and for other studies.

Check with your doctor, and also research the possible side effects of these drugs versus the potential benefits.

Another drug you may want more information on is Xeloda, it targets cancer cells and allegedly leaves healthy cells alone.

RADIATION

If you have breast cancer then you will likely have surgery to remove as much cancer as possible, and then, after some time to heal, you may need radiation to destroy the cancer cells which have been left behind. The radiation will be localized to the breast area, not your whole body.

Before agreeing to radiation, it is critical to meet with a radiation oncologist, a medical doctor who specializes in radiation to treat cancer.

Check-out the following before making your treatment decision:

- **The chance of a recurrence with or without the radiation.**
- **The expected length of each of your radiation treatments.**
- **The number of radiation treatments you will need.**
- **Any side effects you can anticipate from treatment.**
- **What the procedure involves.**
- **What to expect, in general.**
- **Find out if you can have just a SPECIFIC AREA of your breast radiated rather than the whole breast.**

With current technology, you can't have radiation in the same area of your breast if it recurs. You may need a mastectomy for a recurrence, all the more reason to have partial breast radiation if you can.

You will want to feel comfortable with the skills and bedside manner of the radiation oncologist who will order your treatment and with the technicians who give you the radiation.

In this regard, I met a lady named Pat about a year after my mastectomies. She has been a radiation therapist for over 17 years. I asked her to share about her experience with patients' radiation so I could pass along this information to you.

She shared the following in an e-mail: "I can say from experience that there are several different ways to treat breast cancer with radiation, and the course of treatment is designed to suit the medical needs of each patient. Most of my patients come to me after a lumpectomy (and usually chemo first). About 10% (rough estimate) had a single mastectomy (or possibly a double mastectomy), and chemo and still need radiation therapy. Very often women complete the course of treatment (about 6 weeks) with mild side effects that are temporary (skin reddening and fatigue). A few women do have more severe reactions and that often has to do with the patient's anatomy (large pendulous breasts tend to be more prone to skin reactions). I can not recall a woman ending treatment before receiving the prescribed dose, regardless of skin effects. I think breast cancer patients know that the radiation treatment is designed to save their lives and they must do it, so they do. They are all certainly happy to have it over and they are generally very grateful to the therapists who have done what we could to save their lives."

POINTS FROM DR. BARRY:

- **I know women who ended radiation treatment before the prescribed dose was finished.**

Many studies have shown, if you have a lumpectomy followed by radiation, you will decrease your risk of a breast cancer recurrence. You should talk to your doctor and ask him/her about the risk of a recurrence with and without radiation. If you learn you have a 30% higher chance of getting a recurrence if you do not take the radiation understand what this means. If your risk of a recurrence is 10% with the radiation then this means your risk increases by 30% of that 10%, or another 3%, giving you a risk of recurrence of 13% - not the 30% as it may sound like. Be sure to clarify exactly what your doctor means when he/she explains your risk of recurrence with each treatment choice.

Please find out if you can get local radiation, or partial breast radiation, instead of having your whole breast radiated. If it recurs locally (meaning the breast cancer has not spread to other areas of your body) then it usually comes back in the area near where the original breast cancer has been removed. So, you might need more radiation. If your whole breast has already been radiated, you most likely will be unable to receive radiation again, and you may need a mastectomy. Thus, it is best to have your doctor only radiate as much of the area as necessary. Also, the less radiation you receive, the fewer side effects you may have. You still want to ensure you have enough radiation to wipe out as many cancer cells which have been left behind after the lumpectomy or surgery, as possible. This is the whole purpose of the radiation – to destroy the cancer cells.

POINTS FROM DR. BARRY:

- **I have not heard of getting partial breast radiation.**
- **Bracky therapy is radioactive seeds or rods that are temporarily or permanently inserted in the tissue for local radiation. This has been tried with breast cancer but is not presently standard procedure.**
- **Radiation, like a shotgun-fine control, is not yet possible.**

POSSIBLE RISKS AND SIDE EFFECTS FROM RADIATION

- **A portion of your lung may get radiated and cause a cough and/or future lung problems.**
- **Radiation may also increase the risk of lung cancer especially if you are a smoker.**
- **You may get tired, have swelling, redness, and muscle inflammation.**

- If you need to have your lymph nodes under your arm radiated then this may increase your risk of getting lymphedema. (See my section on lymphedema under surgery.)
- If you get radiation on your left breast then you may increase your risk of heart problems.
- Radiation may cause an increased risk of rib fractures. Especially during contact sports or if you have an active lifestyle.

Check with your doctor to see how the added radiation will decrease your risk of getting a breast cancer recurrence. In certain situations it may be necessary to have radiation even after a mastectomy.

POINTS FROM DR. BARRY:

- If you have 4 or more lymph nodes that are positive for cancer or the tumor was close to a margin then you will probably still need radiation even after a mastectomy.

Consider the risk of recurrence for all treatments versus the possible benefit and side effects for each treatment. I believe the best way to make your decision is to assess the risk of recurrence and the chance of survival as opposed to the possible side effects from each treatment.

TREATMENT FOR DCIS

If you or your doctor feel something out of the ordinary in your breast or there is something suspicious on your mammogram then have a biopsy. Don't just have a needle biopsy, actually have the lump or unusual area removed.

POINTS FROM DR. BARRY:

- **A stereotactic needle biopsy can be very accurate.**

Schedule another mammogram a month or two later to ensure all of the calcifications, or other areas of concern, have been removed. (As I've mentioned, in the mammogram I had a few months before my mastectomies I had so many calcifications if they had removed them all, my breasts would have resembled Swiss cheese. They couldn't remove them all with the biopsy, so I opted for the mastectomies.) Make sure to obtain the pathologist's report even if you don't have cancer.

If you do have DCIS (ductal carcinoma in situ) breast cancer then find out:

- **If it is high grade or low grade.**
- **The size of the DCIS.**
- **If necrosis (dead cells) is present.**
- **The size of the clean margin.**
- **If the removed tissue is estrogen-receptor-positive or negative.**
- **If the DCIS is in more than one place.**

POINTS FROM DR. BARRY:

- **Whether it is isolated or multifocal (found in more than one area) DCIS is very important.**

Since it is currently non-invasive, the DCIS cancer should not have spread to your lymph nodes or other parts of your body.

If your removed tissue is estrogen-receptor-positive, it is more sensitive to estrogen. It is then more likely to benefit from the estrogen blocker, Tamoxifen, if you are premenopausal; and an Aromatase Inhibitor and/or Tamoxifen if you are postmenopausal.

If you are diagnosed with a breast cancer other than DCIS, the same questions can be asked. Definitely find out if your cancer is ductal or lobular, and the clinical and pathological staging you are in.

POINTS FROM DR. BARRY:

- **Clinical staging is determined before surgery via exams and tests.**
- **Pathological staging is determined after surgery. The removed tissue is examined.**
- **Sometimes the two are different.**

Breast cancer's origin (meaning where it started) is either ductal or lobular, and it is either non-invasive or invasive. Invasive means it can escape from the ducts and lobules to invade other areas of the breast, lymph nodes, and other parts of the body. Being invasive does not suggest it has already done this, it signifies it is the type of cancer which can spread.)

There are several treatment choices for multifocal DCIS, meaning non-invasive early stage breast cancer found in the milk ducts in multiple places yet hasn't escaped the milk ducts yet.

TREATMENT CHOICES FOR DCIS

- **Wide excision or lumpectomy** which refers to taking out the affected area, and around 1 cm wide, all around the area of normal tissue (a clean margin). (It won't be confirmed as normal tissue until it is biopsied. If a clean border is not achieved then more tissue may need to be removed.)
- **Wide excision or lumpectomy plus radiation.**
- **Wide excision or lumpectomy plus radiation and Tamoxifen** if you are **pre-menopausal** and **Tamoxifen and/or Aramotase Inhibitors** if you are **post-menopausal**.

- o **With regard to the Tamoxifen or Aromatase Inhibitor, find out if your removed tissue is estrogen-receptor-positive or negative.**
- o If it is estrogen-receptor-**negative,** then taking Tamoxifen may not make sense due to risks of side effects for little or no benefit.
- o If it is estrogen-receptor-**positive** then consider taking Tamoxifen or Aramotase Inhibitors because your tissue is stimulated by estrogen.
- o Think about the dangers and benefits of decreasing your risk for cancer in the other breast and/or preventing a recurrence of invasive breast cancer in the breast operated on if you choose these drugs.
- **Mastectomy** - removal of as much of the breast tissue and cells as possible.
  - o You may want to consider a prophylactic removal of the other breast as well since DCIS doubles your risk for breast cancer in the other breast. The larger the area of DCIS, and the more ducts affected by DCIS, the more likely some lymph nodes will also be removed. Select a surgeon skilled enough to do a sentinel node biopsy, so lymph node removal can be kept to a minimum. (See my discussion of sentinel node biopsy and lymphedema.)

I'm sure these are not the treatments you thought would be used for early stage, non-invasive breast cancer. I am still shocked that these are the choices. I agree these treatments seem harsh and drastic for early stage breast cancer, yet, unfortunately, these treatment choices are what Western medicine currently offers.

Many doctors and women suggest saving the breast(s) if at all possible and advocate only performing a mastectomy for women who demand it, or if there is a clear medical advantage for doing so. As a layperson, based on the information I gathered, I realized a bilateral mastectomy would be best for me, even with early stage breast cancer. I wondered, how much poking, prodding, and removing of tissue might I go through if I didn't have them? The mastectomies seemed the surest way to be done with my treatments. You must decide which treatment is best for you.

POINTS FROM DR. BARRY:

- **I look at a breast with multifocal DCIS as a diseased breast and not really salvageable.**
- **If I have a big piece of cheese that has a spot of mold on it such that I can trim it and still have a nice piece to enjoy, I keep it. If, however, the entire hunk of cheese is riddled with mold, by the time I trim it there may not be anything worth saving.**

As I've written earlier, I don't recall my doctors ever discussing a wide excision. Since I had already had two biopsies, and many previous biopsies over the years, these may have been the equivalent of a wide excision. The treatment choices the doctor gave me for my multifocal DCIS were mastectomy, or radiation followed by Tamoxifen.

The goal of your treatment is to prevent the DCIS cancer cells from spreading outside of the duct. If they manage to do this, it then becomes invasive cancer. Unfortunately, we cannot predict when, or in whom this will happen to, or if it will even occur. The good news is if you only have DCIS, your cancer is still non-invasive, and you should not need chemotherapy. Also, as long as your breast cancer remains non-invasive, you will not die from it.

According to <u>Dr. Susan Love's Breast Book</u>, 4th edition, with DCIS the recurrence after mastectomy is 1-2% (both my surgeon and oncologist told me I had a 0-1% chance of a recurrence), and with breast conservation or wide excision there is a 5-10% chance of recurrence. She mentions there is a 1-2% risk of dying from breast cancer for either of these procedures. This didn't make sense to me. I remember my surgeon telling me the studies did not indicate a higher rate of survival after a mastectomy as compared to having the DCIS removed, coupled with radiation and taking Tamoxifen. It would seem if one has a lower rate for a recurrence then the chance of dying from breast cancer would also go down. If you don't get breast cancer again then how do you die of it?

POINTS FROM DR. BARRY:

- **The 0-1% versus the 1-2% statistic cited above is not statistically significant. In a large enough study you might not find a difference.**

It seems reasonable that if you have a wide excision along with radiation you would decrease your risk for recurrence and invasive breast cancer, as compared to just a wide excision.

You may decrease your risk for recurrence even more if you add Tamoxifen to the wide excision and radiation. If you do get a recurrence while taking Tamoxifen, the Tamoxifen will decrease the risk that the breast cancer is invasive. Yet again, explore the potential side effects of taking Tamoxifen (see Tamoxifen discussion) and seriously weigh them against the possible benefits you may or may not receive.

With the screening tests now available to detect breast cancer and the improvement in treatments, it seems incredible that women still die from breast cancer. Remember, early detection saves lives. Sadly, this phrase doesn't always include saving our breasts.

POINTS FROM DR. BARRY:

- **I am pretty fatalistic about breast cancer. With Stage 0 or I breast cancer, I feel that logically there is good reason to believe that surgical excision can be curative.**
- **With Stage III or IV breast cancer it really depends more on the intrinsic characteristics of the individual tumor as to what the survival will be. Chemotherapy/radiation may prolong a patient's life but at a cost of side effects. Some tolerate the side effects better than others.**

COMPLIMENTARY <u>BUT NOT</u> ALTERNATIVE TREATMENTS

By complimentary treatment, I mean anything you may want to do to help your mind and body beyond traditional Western medicine. Whatever you do, do not let these choices prevent you from having your traditional Western medicine treatment. These suggestions are meant to be in addition to your doctor's recommended treatment, **not** to stand alone. With that said, what you are trying to achieve is a positive mental attitude. If any of these can help, utilize them. If not, then disregard these recommendations.

Things to try:

- **yoga,**
- **be hypnotized,**
- **pray,**
- **become more involved in your religion and the people at your place of worship,**
- **have faith,**
- **go to a therapist,**
- **meditate,**

- visualize being well, laugh,
- be with fun people,
- get healing rocks like an amethyst,
- eat right, though check with your doctor before making any diet changes,
- exercise - join a gym or an exercise group,
- find an exercise partner,
- join a walking group,
- have a massage,
- learn relaxation techniques,
- do things that relax you, whatever that means for you (i.e. dancing, quilting, mountain climbing, swimming, traveling, reading…),
- schedule a facial,
- indulge in a foot massage,
- try acupuncture,
- see an herbalist and take special vitamins and herbs. (Check this out first with your doctor.)

TREATMENTS OF THE NEAR FUTURE

During the next decade hopeful drugs which "silence" specific genes will be coming out on the market. They may be capable of halting the specific genes linked to breast cancer and mutations from doing their vile work.

There are six to nine ductal systems in the female breast. I believe what occurs in the milk ducts, and their relationship to estrogen is key to discovering what causes and/or can prevent breast cancer.

We need to know what happens in the human body so we can stop cancer cells from forming and/or from spreading and becoming more destructive. Maybe it could be similar to how a flu shot creates a mild case of the flu; a mild case of breast cancer could be given which will not become aggressive.

POINTS FROM DR. BARRY:

- ### The flu shot approach is an interesting idea.

Imagine if it could be like Ms. Pac Man where something is given to women which goes into their ducts and chases down the little dots, cancer cells, and eats them. Something must be invented to prevent breast cancer, provide a mild dose of breast cancer as mentioned earlier, and/or effectively stop breast cancer's progression.

In writing this book I have realized there is a plethora of research being done on breast cancer. It has me wonder if there is an agency to review all of the studies and check for the common threads which may provide a cure or treatment for breast cancer.

There is such an agency. If you want more reading then you can go to www.ctsu.ox.ac.uk/projects/ebctcg to see the Early Breast Cancer Trialists Collaborative Group (EBCTCG) report of all randomized clinical trials regarding early stage breast cancer.

In reading some of the scientific studies, I realize I do not completely understand the scientific jargon. I can only make a layman's interpretation of what is being said, so I'm certain to be missing some interesting points.

E. HOW TO MAKE YOUR TREATMENT CHOICE

Depending on your breast cancer diagnosis and your prognosis, you may or may not be given the choice of which treatment to take. Your Oncologist is usually the doctor who lays out your treatment choices, and he/she may decide what is best for you.

In my situation, they'd found DCIS in several areas of my breast. I had several treatment choices. None of my doctors suggested which treatment to take, they only requested I "do something." They left the treatment choice to me. You might be presented with the same challenge, so I have some advice below.

POINTERS ON MAKING YOUR TREATMENT DECISION

- As difficult as it is, try to take emotion out of your treatment decision.
- Be as objective as you possibly can be under the circumstances.
- Talk to your doctors and find out what stage breast cancer you have.
- Ask them what your treatment options are and the pluses and minuses for each choice.
- Ask your doctors what your chance of recurrence is with each treatment option.
- If you are of Ashkenazi Jewish descent, or have a few close blood relatives who have had breast cancer, ovarian cancer or melanomas; then have the BRCA1 and BRCA2 gene counseling to decide about taking the gene mutation blood/ saliva test.
- If you are positive for the gene mutation then consider having a double mastectomy. Depending on your age and whether you still want to give birth to your own children, consider having your ovaries removed.
- AGAIN, PLEASE do your own research to choose the treatment which is right for YOU!
- If you are diagnosed with breast cancer, YOU must carefully analyze your alternatives. Please choose the treatment which gives you the best chance of survival with the least chance for recurrence while considering the possible side effects of each option.
- Ask your doctors many questions. Never be afraid to speak up. You are the patient, and your doctor is there to serve YOU.

POINTS FROM DR. BARRY:

- Yes, ask your doctor's questions but keep in mind how overwhelmed you are.
- Take notes.
- Have someone go with you and let them take notes.
- Ask the doctor if you can tape record the visit.
- Patients have a tendency to not get the information the first or second go around. Answering the same question over and over again can overwhelm the doctor.
- Remember, you are not their only patient.
- Doing your own research is also helpful.

- **Talk to women who have had each treatment.**
- Do research on the internet by using good sources. (See some of the helpful sites I used at the end of this book.)
- Read this book.
- Read <u>Dr. Susan Love's Breast Book</u> by Susan M. Love, M.D. with Karen Lindsey. Buy her most recent one which at this writing is the 4th Edition.
- You may want to contact Dr. Love for a second opinion regarding your diagnosis and your treatment choice.
  - o (I regret not contacting and seeing Dr. Love before my mastectomies. She lives here in California and may have had other choices for me. At minimum, she could have used my breast history and pathology to help other women. She has dedicated her life and career to studying the breasts and knows more about breast cancer than I do and most likely, a majority of the doctors as well. When reading

her book, it isn't necessary to read all 620 pages.
Go right to the areas which pertain to your
situation.)

- There is so much information on breast cancer, you may feel overwhelmed. You can't get through all of it. Simply gather enough information, and read through what you can, to make an informed decision.
- I believe the key to surviving breast cancer is to find it early and then have the right treatment for your age, ethnic background, and your risk factors.
- Do not let your fears take over. Do whatever you need to remain calm.
- Take care of yourself.
- Be good to yourself.
- Do not blame yourself for having breast cancer.
- Do not let fear get in the way of your need to focus, research, and make some important decisions. It is critical that you know your options, so you can make an educated decision about which treatment is right for you.
- You don't need to be an expert on all types of cancer or all breast cancers, yet at minimum, find out what type of breast cancer you have and learn as much as you can about your particular situation.
- Get accurate information from reliable sources.
- Consider your options and treatment choices, then figure out what makes the most sense for you.
- Reflect on the length of your expected survival with each treatment option as opposed to the side effects of the treatment.
- Prepare for your breast cancer treatment choice as if it is the biggest test or research project of your life. In all honesty, it may be the biggest choice of your life because your life may be at stake.
- Ask your Doctor about clinical trials for your type of cancer, if this seems right. I have never participated in a

clinical trial nor has it ever been mentioned by any of my doctors. You can learn more about finding a clinical trial at: www.cancer.gov (click on the box near the top of the screen) or 1-800-4-Cancer.
- A second opinion from another doctor is a wise alternative.

POINTS FROM DR. BARRY:

- **Yes, second opinions are great but if you are on your 5th "second opinion" you may be having problems dealing with the reality of your situation. When all of the doctors are basically saying the same thing, it only delays your therapy, so be reasonable.**

- Know as much as you can about the potential risks and side effects for all surgeries, anesthesia, procedures, medications, and treatments you may receive and evaluate these risks alongside the potential benefit for each treatment choice.
- Ask your doctors questions and express your concerns and desires.
- Imagine your best friend must make this decision. What would you suggest she do?
- Try to take yourself out of the equation as much as possible.
- What makes the most sense for the given factual scenario at hand?
- Whatever decision you make is the right one for you as you must live with it.

There are so many factors involved with breast cancer. You did not cause it by stress, poor diet, being overweight, or not exercising enough. However, I do believe some of these factors may contribute to having it. You may not have brought about your breast cancer but an unhealthy lifestyle may have played a role in it.

If you are diagnosed with breast cancer, be thankful. I know this sounds strange. Yet I'm fairly certain you wouldn't want to have it and not know about it. Obviously, you would rather not have it at all. But if for some reason you do have it, be thankful for your diagnosis. Life after breast cancer can be invigorating. Most survivors I have talked to really understand the value of life. They've learned to appreciate what they have rather than what they may have lost.

Women should not die of breast cancer with so many treatment options available. It is so important to fully-participate in seeking the right choice for you. First you must be diligent with caring for your breasts as I've discussed throughout the book. If you are diagnosed, you want this to be done as early as possible.

Hopefully you won't need to make a breast cancer treatment decision. If you must make this decision, have a game plan and do what is right for you.

There are many distinctions to take into account for each type of breast cancer. Each woman has her own needs and circumstances so make sure you discuss your optimal treatments with your doctor.

DOCTOR COMPATIBILITY

Thoroughly research all of your doctors, including your surgeon, oncologist, radiation oncologist, and even the anesthesiologist. Obtain referrals from friends, family, nursing staff, or other patients. Interview the doctors to learn their professional background and experience-levels, so you are fully-aware of their knowledge and skills. You will form important relationships with the different doctors and medical people involved in your breast cancer journey. Essentially, they become your healing community which you rely upon for support. You will want to feel comfortable talking with them, and certainly you want to trust your medical providers.

Remember you are entrusting these people with your life. Never feel embarrassed about asking questions and/or changing doctors if you find it necessary to do so. Consider how we readily interview someone before we hire him/her to work for us. We need to do the same with the doctors whom we trust with our care.

Take charge of your breast cancer diagnosis and your decisions to your fullest abilities. Think about the profile of a doctor you want to work with ahead of time. Ensure he/she can meet your needs. Some questions to ask yourself are: Do you prefer a doctor to make most or all of your decisions without sharing much information? Would you like a doctor to be the ultimate decision-maker yet also keep you informed? Would you rather have someone who gives you information and allows you to make your own decisions? Do you need a doctor who provides you information and helps guide you while being supportive? Do you prefer someone who is compassionate and caring?

Since I did not think my surgeon and oncologist gave me enough information, I began doing extensive research on my own which led me to write this book. I doubt you'll want to spend over three years researching about breast cancer as I have. Hopefully, you will have capable doctors who make the best choices for you. I admit I can be somewhat of a control freak and prefer to make my own important decisions. To do this, one must have as much accurate information as possible. However, the investigative process can not go on forever. At some point we must make our final decisions and move forward. Deadlines help. With early stage breast cancers it isn't necessary to make an immediate decision. I recommend you allow a few weeks or a month to absorb the fact that you actually have breast cancer. Then begin your inquiry, surround yourself with the right medical team, and finally, make your decision.

STANDARD OF CARE/GUIDELINE

For a pretty straightforward guideline or standard of care regarding cancer in general and specifically the STANDARD OF CARE for different types of breast cancer, please see the National Comprehensive Cancer Network, NCCN, website at www.nccn.org. Click on "NCCN Clinical Practice Guidelines in Oncology" and then go to your particular type of breast cancer. You can also go into "patients" and then "guidelines." The first site is designed more for medical professionals yet both seemed easy to navigate and understand.

DISTINCTIONS

Treatments may differ for premenopausal or postmenopausal women. They may also be varied for estrogen-receptor-positive or negative women and for women with the BRCA1 or BRCA2 gene mutation. Women who have cancer in their lymph nodes will also be given different treatment choices. These distinctions must be taken into account by you and your doctors.

There is not one breast cancer treatment for all women. A woman's individual situation must be evaluated before she is given treatment. Factors such as a woman's age, current health situation aside from having breast cancer, as well as the benefits, risks, and side effects involved in each treatment choice, must all be taken into consideration.

PREMENOPAUSAL WOMEN

If you are PREMENOPAUSAL then your ovaries are the main source of your estrogen production. You can block the breasts' source of estrogen by cutting off their supply of estrogen from the ovaries. This can be accomplished by the surgical removal of the ovaries called an oopherectomy, radiation to the ovaries, or through hormonal manipulation via hormone therapy. (Again, do not confuse this with Hormone Replacement Therapy (HRT), a controversial treatment, which may be used for postmenopausal symptoms.)

If you have the BRCA1 or BRCA2 gene mutation then depending on your age and if you don't want to give birth to a child, you can consider having your ovaries removed (an oopherectomy) to decrease your risk of ovarian and breast cancer. Keep in mind the oopherectomy will accelerate menopause.

When premenopausal your ovaries create estrogen. After becoming postmenopausal, if you still have your ovaries, they produce other hormones which can be made into estrogen. You are more likely to benefit from either removing your ovaries, or blocking their production of estrogen or other hormones earlier on, IF your breast tissue is estrogen-receptor-positive. The less estrogen which flows into a breast sensitive to it, the better. Keep in mind you may develop other problems in your body due to not having enough estrogen. Discuss all potential side effects with your doctor before selecting a treatment choice. See: www.breastcancer.org/treatment/hormonal/ ovary_removal.jsp (an underscore after the word "ovary") for more information about "ovarian shutdown or removal."

Drugs such as Zoladex which is the same as Goserelin can cause a temporary, reversible menopause which may be helpful in fighting breast cancer. Studies have shown that even a two or three year decrease in estrogen production decreased the risk for a breast cancer recurrence and may provide the same benefit as actually removing the ovaries.

PREMENOPAUSAL women may need to BLOCK ESTROGEN from the breasts, if they are estrogen-receptor-positive, with a drug such as Tamoxifen. (See my discussion below regarding Estrogen-receptor-positive breast tissue.)

POSTMENOPAUSAL WOMEN

IF you are POSTMENOPAUSAL then the ovaries are no longer the main source of your estrogen production. Thus, blocking your ovaries production of estrogen via drugs, surgery, or radiation may be of little or no value to you.

A postmenopausal woman's ovaries are now creating other hormones such as testosterone and androstenedione. These hormones get turned into estrogen by an ENZYME called AROMATASE. Aromatase generates most of the estrogen in postmenopausal women. You may have heard of something called Aromatase Inhibitors. These relatively new drugs could be beneficial for postmenopausal women. Aromatase Inhibitors work by blocking or inactivating aromatase, the enzyme which converts hormones into estrogen in post-menopausal women.

Some studies have shown that the breasts of postmenopausal women with breast cancer have the enzyme aromatase in them. It is thought the aromatase helps supply the breast with estrogen. Thus, it makes sense to take an Aromatase Inhibitor to halt the aromatase from entering the breast and creating estrogen.

The Aromatase Inhibitors Anastrozole (Arimidex) and Letrozole (Femara) BLOCK the aromatase enzyme on a reversible basis. Another aromatase inhibitor, Exemestane (Aromasin) permanently inactivates the aromatase enzyme.

Even though these drugs are somewhat new on the market, they have had impressive results in studies on POSTMENOPAUSAL WOMEN WITH ESTROGEN-POSITIVE metastatic disease and other POSTMENOPAUSAL WOMEN WITH ESTROGEN-POSITIVE breast cancer. Note, all of these women had tissue/lumps which were ESTROGEN-RECEPTOR- POSITIVE meaning they were sensitive to estrogen.

Since Tamoxifen can only be taken for five years, postmenopausal women may consider taking one of these Aromatase Inhibitors when they finish Tamoxifen, especially if they are at a high risk of recurrence. Studies are also underway to find out if POSTMENOPAUSAL WOMEN WHO ARE ESTROGEN-RECEPTOR-POSITIVE can benefit by taking an Aromatase Inhibitor alone without first taking Tamoxifen.

IS YOUR BREAST TISSUE ESTROGEN-RECEPTOR- POSITIVE?

You MUST FIND OUT if your tissue removed during a biopsy, lumpectomy, wide excision or mastectomy is **ESTROGEN-RECEPTOR-POSITIVE OR NEGATIVE.**

No one ever told me if my tissue which had been removed during my many biopsies or my mastectomies had tested estrogen-receptor-positive or negative. How would I have known about the testing? One would think this would be standard procedure since the results help women make informed decisions about which treatments to choose.

(Long after my mastectomies I found out my removed tissue was estrogen-receptor-positive.)

I really didn't understand this significance until doing my research for this book, after my mastectomies. To derive the maximum benefit from Tamoxifen, my tissue needed to be estrogen-receptor-positive, meaning estrogen greatly affected my breast tissue.

Had my tests shown me to be estrogen-receptor-negative, then I might not have received any benefit from Tamoxifen. Why take a drug with so many possible side effects when one may not have any benefit from it?

If you recall, Tamoxifen is used to **block** estrogen from getting into the breast. If your breast tissue/lump isn't sensitive to estrogen, then you most likely will not benefit from preventing the estrogen from entering your breast.

YOU MUST have the lump/tissue which is removed during your biopsy, lumpectomy, or wide excision analyzed to know if it is estrogen-receptor-negative or positive, sensitive, to estrogen to make an informed treatment choice. Do not assume this is standard protocol as it should be.

MAKE SURE your tissue is tested for its reaction to ESTROGEN and obtain the results BEFORE you make a treatment choice, so you can make your best decision.

If your removed tissue is **estrogen-receptor-positive**, you may benefit from taking Tamoxifen if you are premenopausal, or Tamoxifen and/or Aromatase Inhibitors if you are postmenopausal, by decreasing the risk for breast cancer in your other breast and/or a recurrence in the breast diagnosed with cancer. As always, consider your options, risks, and potential benefits before making your decision.

If your breast tissue **is estrogen-receptor-negative** then neither Tamoxifen or Aromatase Inhibitors may help you. So, it doesn't make much sense to take them with the side effects and risks of other problems when you would receive little or no benefit.

Postmenopausal women often have tumors which are estrogen-receptor-positive and **premenopausal** women generally have tumors which are estrogen-receptor-negative. This could be due to our fluctuations in hormones. We may experience variations after menopause than before. It could be the cumulative effect of all of the hormone fluctuations over our lifetime which has us be more likely to have estrogen-receptor-positive tumors during our postmenopausal years.

THE BRCA1 or BRCA2 GENE MUTATION

If you are diagnosed with breast cancer at an early age (before age 40), have a family history of breast cancer, colon cancer, melanomas, and/or prostate cancer then schedule gene counseling and discuss the BRCA1 or BRCA2 gene mutation tests. The tests require a blood draw or the giving of your salivia, both very easy to do.

If you are diagnosed with atypical cells, DCIS or any breast cancer, and it is determined you have the BRCA1 or BRCA2 gene mutation, then seriously consider a bilateral mastectomy (removal of both of your breasts) and/or an oopherectomy (removal of your ovaries).

Please see my previous, lengthy discussion of the BRCA1 and BRCA2 gene mutation and test in my section entitled "**Breast Cancer Screening: Genetics-The BRCA1 and BRCA2 Gene Mutation.**"

FOLLOW-UP

Make sure your doctors discuss a follow-up plan with you. This should take place **before** you select your treatment. I know dealing with your breast cancer can be overwhelming. You may want to just put it behind you, yet it is critical to do all you can to avoid a recurrence and/or to find a recurrence as early as possible.

Your follow-up doctor will be your oncologist, radiation oncologist and/or your surgeon. You will want to have a positive, comfortable relationship with them. Make sure you know who will be on your follow-up medical team. Ensure your doctors check-in with how you are healing mentally and physically as well as monitor for signs of a recurrence in your scars, breasts, lymph nodes, and body.

It took me almost one year and a half after my mastectomies to develop a follow-up plan. I found this very frustrating. I encourage you to talk with your doctors before and during treatments about who will work with you on an ongoing basis. Ask them what your follow-up will entail.

SUPPORT

It is important to have a strong support system of friends, family, neighbors, and co-workers during your entire breast cancer experience.

Support Groups

You may find it helpful to connect with a support group specifically for women with breast cancer. There are many groups available. You can check with your doctors or go online to find one near you. You may want one with women who have **a similar diagnosis.** I didn't join a support group because I feared what I might learn from them. I didn't want to be around women who were dying of breast cancer.

Also, I had enough support from my family and friends, so I did not need an outside source. If you need a support group or counseling, by all means go for it. You can ask your doctor or search on the internet for one near you. Do whatever will help bring as much ease as possible to your life. Be willing to reach out for help during your breast cancer journey.

OTHER THINGS TO CONSIDER

A RECURRENCE

- **The longer you go without a recurrence, the better your chances of not having one.**
- **If you go 10 years without a recurrence, then you most likely will not have one.**
- **Do all you can to avoid a recurrence.**
- **Eat right; exercise; don't drink much alcohol; don't become overweight; have follow-ups with your doctors; and choose the best medical treatment to get rid of your breast cancer and offer you the least chance of a recurrence.**
- **Ask your doctors, particularly your oncologist, for the likelihood of a recurrence with each treatment choice you consider.**

One of the biggest factors regarding survival after breast cancer is the length of time before a recurrence. The longer you can go without a recurrence, the better it is for your longevity.

I believe the best treatment is the one with the best chance for survival and the least potential for recurrence, while taking into account the side effects of the treatment. It is vital to do whatever you can to prevent breast cancer from recurring or spreading to other parts of your body.

A LOCAL RECURRENCE

- **A LOCAL recurrence is when breast cancer cells return to the breast area.**
- **If the local recurrence is an early stage non-invasive breast cancer, then it may only be some cancer cells left behind during your previous treatment. You require surgery to get rid of this newly found cancer.**

- If it is an invasive breast cancer, then you will need further treatment to stop the cancer from spreading.

A LOCAL RECURRENCE AFTER BREAST CONSERVATION TREATMENT

- Most recurrences occur in the same area as the original cancer and often appear three to four years after your initial treatment.
- If you had radiation before, you may be unable to have it again in the same area of the breast. Thus, you may need a mastectomy.
- If the cancer shows up in a different area of the breast which had breast cancer before, it could be a new, primary breast cancer and not a recurrence.
- If you had partial radiation to a specific part of the breast during your prior treatment, you may be able to have it again in the same breast in another area. Talk to your doctors about this if you are inclined to do more radiation rather than have a mastectomy.

A LOCAL RECURRENCE AFTER A MASTECTOMY

- If you have a recurrence after a mastectomy, it will most likely be in or near the surgical scar, chest wall, or under the skin.
- A recurrence reportedly feels like a hard knuckle under your skin. 90% of them occur within the first five years after a mastectomy. After you've passed the five year milestone you can breathe easier; however, it is still important

to pay attention to your body for any signs of a recurrence.

- If you have implants they should not interfere with finding the recurrence because it usually shows up in front of the implant.
- If you do have a LOCAL recurrence (meaning it isn't in other parts of your body), then you may need the lump removed with follow-up radiation if this area of the breast has not had radiation before.

METASTATIC/DISTANT RECURRENCE

- This means the breast cancer has spread to an organ outside of the breast.
- Unfortunately, it may not be curable.
- Only a small percentage of women will be cured. You can be one of them.
- It is possible to go into remission for 20 years or more.
- It depends upon where the breast cancer has extended to. The chances are greater for survival if the cancer has spread to the bone or the skin, as opposed to, the lung or liver.

SYMPTOMS AND WHAT THEY MAY MEAN:

- Constant bone pain which persists for a week or two even while you are sleeping can indicate the breast cancer has infiltrated into your bones. See your doctor as you will probably need a bone scan.
- Shortness of breath and/or a chronic cough can signify the cancer is now in your lungs. This is not good news. Of the women who die from breast cancer, 60-70% of them had breast cancer

which moved into their lungs. If you have these symptoms, please see your doctor for a chest x-ray.

- **Loss of appetite, weight loss (without dieting), nausea and stomach problems can mean the cancer is now in your liver. See your doctor and get a blood test and/or CT scan, MRI and PET scan.**
- **Headaches and a change in vision may indicate the cancer has spread into your brain and/or spinal cord. See your doctor and have a CAT scan or MRI.**

Be relentless. If you have any of these symptoms go to your doctor for a thorough examination. Be tested to ensure your cancer has not moved to any other areas of your body.

CLINICAL TRIALS/STUDIES

You can participate in a study which pertains to your particular type of breast cancer and/or treatment choice.

Visit the National Cancer Institute's website at www.cancer.gov and click on "breast cancer" and then "clinical trials" to see a wide assortment of trials you may qualify for. You can also call the National Cancer Institute at 1-800-4-Cancer. Obtain a list of clinical trials at www.nccn.org which is the National Comprehensive Cancer Network or NCCN. Click on "patients" and then on "clinical trials." Definitely discuss clinical trials with your doctor and obtain their approval before you participate in any trials. Trials often involve testing a drug or treatment for its effectiveness on a certain group of people. Be sure to research the potential benefits, side effects, and risks before you participate in the study.

I didn't know about these studies before my mastectomies. In retrospect, there were some studies I could have participated in with little effort which would have provided helpful information to the people conducting the study.

If you want more information then visit: www.ctsu.ox.ac.uk/projects/ebctcg to read the Early Breast Cancer Trialists Collaborative Group's (EBCTCG) report of all randomized clinical trials regarding early stage breast cancer. Since there are so many studies, the group seems to only update them every four or five years. I noticed a summary of data from 2000 and then again in 2005/2006. This compilation is geared more toward other scientists than us. Yet it is helpful to know there is a group assembling studies for other scientists to look at.

New trials are underway with drugs which may help with metastatic breast cancer. A drug called Trastuzumab is thought to block the Her-2/neu oncogene similar to how Tamoxifen prevents estrogen from reaching the breast.

Another drug Bevacizumab is being tested to find out if it can target the new blood vessels being formed which feed the cancer and encourage its growth.

IF you have **metastic breast cancer,** then it may be in your best interest to join a clinical trial since the treatments for metastic breast cancer have not been studied as much as the ones for local/non-metastic breast cancer. Please go to: www.cancer.gov which is the National Cancer Institute's website for some clinical trials which may benefit you. Again, check with your doctor before agreeing to participate in any clinical trial or study. Also, consider joining a support group with other women whose breast cancer has metastasized.

TISSUE BANKS

Dr. Love recommends depositing your breast tissue in a tissue bank before any surgical procedure to your breast, whether a biopsy, wide excision, breast reduction, or mastectomy. I asked my surgeon, Dr. X, if my breast tissue had been placed in a tissue bank. She replied, "No," with a long, blank stare as if I'd lost my wits to ask such a question. I'm not aware of any tissue banks, yet do ask your doctor and research them if you think it makes sense.

I would have appreciated knowing about tissue banks for breast tissue before my biopsies and mastectomies. Having someone study and learn something from my tissue would have been reassuring. If nothing else, it would have been helpful for the doctors to use it to compare what they missed in the ultrasound, needle biopsy, mammogram, stereotactic biopsies, and physical examination versus what had actually been found by the pathologists after they removed and examined my breasts. This could have been a tremendous learning experience. To my knowledge, they did nothing with my breast tissue after any of the procedures.

I found some tissue banks on the internet. I know nothing about them so proceed with caution. Be certain they are not a scam before you work with them. Hopefully, your doctor will have more information for you than mine had for me.

HOW DOES BREAST CANCER GROW AND SPREAD?

If breast cancer cells escape from the breast duct they must have their own blood supply to continue growing, otherwise they will die. A tumor may be able to get to 2mm before it needs more blood vessels to provide it with food for growth. It is thought that a protein called VEGF (vascular endothelial growth factor) is secreted by the cancer which then attaches to existing blood vessels and orders them to produce more blood vessels. This VEGF may be the same protein secreted when you are injured and must create new blood vessels to heal your injury. I may be stretching it here, yet the many biopsies I had may have sent a signal indicating I'd been injured. Thus, proteins or cells responded to heal the area stimulating breast cancer. Could this be feasible?

My dad died of cancer six years ago. His large cancerous tumor had become the size of a volleyball in his abdomen. Two weeks later he died. They gave him blood transfusions to strengthen him for surgery. I am not sure if the new blood fed his cancer or not. What I do know is after they opened him up to perform the surgery, the surgeon later told us he could not do the surgery because the cancer had attached to all of his major organs. He would have bled to death on the surgery table if he attempted to remove this tumor. So my thoughts are his cancer produced VEGF which then created many new blood cells through *angiogenesis (angio*=vessels *and* genesis=growth (angiogenesis means the growth of blood vessels). The more blood vessels there are, the greater the blood supply to feed the cancer. Subsequently these blood vessels wrapped around his major organs making it impossible to remove the tumor.

I imagine all cancers must create a blood supply so they can grow. The more you bleed during surgery, the worse your cancer may be due to the increased blood supply from the cancer itself. This blood supply allows the cancer to grow uncontrollably.

Even DCIS, early stage breast cancer, still in the duct and not yet invasive, may be producing an increased number of blood vessels around the outside of the duct. What exactly is this early stage breast cancer doing? The DCIS is secreting *angiogenic* proteins like VEGF to create new blood vessels that are possibly preparing for a future departure out of the duct and into the blood and body. This goes back to the not knowing of in whom or when DCIS will be able to break out of the duct and become invasive cancer. DCIS certainly seems to have the capacity to spread. As of yet we do not know what triggers this mellow DCIS cancer to transform to invasive cancer.

A test to detect VEGF levels in the blood or milk ducts would be extremely beneficial. If one existed, most likely higher levels would indicate more blood vessels underway which would soon allow the cancer to escape and multiply throughout the body. This would help women with DCIS to know whether or not they must take serious measures to get rid of their DCIS.

In my own situation, I had two biopsies within a week which did not bleed much. New blood vessels may have developed to heal my surgical wounds. About a month later I had a stereotactic biopsy which I'd expected to be less intrusive than my other biopsies. Instead I bled a lot and even formed a hematoma.

Hopefully, the drug Bevacizumab will prove effective in stopping the VEGF protein thus, preventing *angiogenesis,* the production of new blood vessels which permit the cancer to spread.

THE FUTURE

There is much to be learned about the function of the breast ducts, especially when they are not breastfeeding. In studying breasts, scientists may discover what causes cancer to start in the milk ducts. This may help prevent breast cancer or reverse it. Researchers may develop a pill or an injection for the breasts capable of destroying only the cancer cells rather than the good cells, without the need for surgery.

Hopefully, more targeted therapies customized for each woman's hormonal composition and genetic make-up will become available. Scientists may discover more effective ways to control, prevent, or even reverse breast cancer to make breast cells "normal."

Can scientists learn how to stop VEGF proteins from creating new blood vessels when cancer is involved? Let's support this research, if the opportunity exists. This would make a tremendous difference for eradicating breast cancer and all cancers.

WHAT I HOPE THAT YOU WILL DO

- **Learn as much as you can about breast cancer.**
- **Be mindful of the factors which may contribute to your getting breast cancer and practice self-care.**
- **Use the screening tools currently available to detect breast cancer and if you are diagnosed, find it in its early stages.**
- **If you do have breast cancer, know your treatment choices and make an informed decision. Weigh the possibility of a**

recurrence and the chance of survival against all possible side effects for each treatment choice.

- **If you do the above, then I have been successful in getting my ideas and information across to you.**

My thoughts for a healthy and fulfilling life are with you.

Andrea

AFTERWARD

Four years have passed since my diagnosis of early stage breast cancer. Thankfully, I am still cancer free. I believe breast cancer is behind me. I am healthier, more muscular, and both physically and mentally stronger than I have ever been. I am so grateful for all I have, including my firm, reconstructed breasts. My handsome son, Andrew, is now 5 and my beautiful daughter, Gabby, is 13. The years go by quickly.

If you are diagnosed with breast cancer, be thankful. Although this may seem strange, I am fairly certain you would rather know about it so you can take immediate action. Obviously, you would rather not have breast cancer at all. Yet if you do have it, know life after breast cancer can be invigorating. Most survivors I have talked with really understand the value of life. They've learned to appreciate what they have rather than what they may have lost.

Women should not die from breast cancer with so many treatment options and screening tests available. Remember, early detection saves lives, not necessarily breasts. Please be diligent with caring for your breasts as I've discussed throughout the book. If you are diagnosed with breast cancer, do not panic. Follow the guidance I have provided you in this book and make the treatment choice which is right for you. In summary, select the treatment which offers you the best chance of survival with the least chance of a recurrence. Always weigh in the possible side effects from each treatment choice.

I wish you the very best of health. Feel free to contact me at Andrea964@aol.com. Please see my website www.thriveandsurvive. net

Andrea

LIST OF RESOURCES:

Internet sites:

www.thriveandsurvive.net Andrea's breast cancer website.

http://www.ncbi.nlm.nih.gov/pubmed/12927427 Regarding the million women study in the UK.

www.getbcfacts.com/treatment/questionsfor.asp A great list of questions to ask your various doctors and specialists.

www.getbcfacts.com/treatment/team.asp- Brief descriptions of the health care professionals you may need to see.

www.webmd.com/breast cancer- Helpful articles and information. Sign up for their email list and they will send you breast cancer updates.

http://www.cancer.org/docroot/CRI/content/CRI__2_6x_Exercises_ After_Breast_Surgery.asp - (There is an underscore (_)after CRI and all of the blank spots above). Exercises after breast surgery and radiation.

www.cancer.gov and a study NSABP B24

www.paptestforthebreast.com and www.neomatrix.com Discusses the Halo Naf breast screening exam.

http://www.cancer.gov/cancertopics/aromatase-inhibitors- Aromatase Inhibitors lower the amount of estrogen and block the growth of tumors.

http://www.cancer.gov/cancertopics/treatment/breast/aromatase-inhibitors0307 Aromatase Inhibitors lower the amount of estrogen and block the growth of tumors.

http://www.cancer.gov/cancertopics/breast-cancer-surgery-choices - A site by the National Cancer Institute which helps women with early stage breast cancer to make a treatment choice.

American Cancer Society (1 800-227-2345 or www.cancer.org) or the National Breast and Cervical Cancer Early Detection Program (1- 888-842-6355) or www.cdc.gov/cancer/nbccedp For low cost mammograms.

http://www.4woman.gov/faq/earlybc.htm by The National Women's Health Information Center is very helpful. The 10 page article entitled, "Early Stage Breast Cancer: A Patient and Doctor Dialogue" defined terminology and answered many questions. You can also call (1-800-994-9662).

Books:

Dr. Susan Love's Breast Book by Susan M. Love, M.D. with Karen Lindsey. Request the most recent edition which at this writing is the 4th Edition. This book is the bible of breast cancer and is a must read!

My daughter GABBY'S PAPER

(She was 11 when she wrote this.) 1/27/08

WHAT YOU NEED TO KNOW ABOUT BREAST CANCER

One out of every eight girls born in the United States of Aerica today will be inflicted by a potentially fatal disease that has no cure. The most common women's cancer in America is breast cancer. How would you feel if your daughter, sister or mother was diagnosed with breast cancer? Breast cancer is a common disease in women and is yet to be cured.

Early detection of breast cancer saves lives. Breast cancer is an uncontrolled, potentially deadly division of cells in the breast. In women, it is the most common type of cancer and the second most deadly cancer. Breast cancer usually begins with the formation of a small confined tumor and is very treatable if it is found early. If not found early, breast cancer can be deadly.

A lot of things can cause breast cancer and we have to be aware of them. Researchers think that the greater a woman's level of estrogen, the more vulnerable she is to breast cancer. Estrogen tells cells to divide. The more cells that divide, the more likely they are to be abnormal and possibly cancerous. High fat diets may also cause breast cancer. Obesity and more than a few drinks of alcohol a day can also cause breast cancer. These are just a few of the many things that can cause breast cancer.

Every woman is at risk for getting breast cancer sometime in her life. Women whose mother, sister, or daughter has had breast cancer are two to three times more likely to get breast cancer. Some instances of familial breast cancer occur when there is a mutation of two genes called BRCA1 and BRCA2. Only one in 200 people carry the gene mutation and having it does not ensure they will get breast cancer, but, having the gene mutation does increase the person's chance of getting breast cancer. A woman's risk increases if she starts menstruating before age 12 or has her first child after age 30. Women's risks decrease if they nurse their children and the longer the nursing the better protection against breast cancer. These are some of the many risk factors of breast cancer.

Symptoms of breast cancer can vary. Some are more serious than others. Some symptoms include painless lumps, areas of tissue that feel sore or hard when pressed, and persistent pain under the armpit. Doctors recommend annual mammograms for women over 40 years old. A mammogram is an x-ray that can detect many cancers before they can be felt. While there can be many symptoms associated with breast cancer, thankfully, there are ways to help detect it early.

Treatments for breast cancer vary depending on how early it is detected. A lumpectomy is used for small lumps. The surgeon removes the cancerous lump and a margin of the tissue around it. Then the breast may be treated with radiation to kill stray cancerous cells and the patient may have to take Tamoxifen or other medication. If the cancer is large or has spread or the person is afraid of a recurrence, the whole breast may be removed. In a modified radical mastectomy the lymph nodes are removed from the armpit. Lymph nodes are small masses of tissue that help the body fight disease. Tamoxifen is a drug taken orally for prevention and treatment of breast cancer. Chemotherapy is another treatment that attempts to kill cancer cells. The higher the stage of breast cancer, the more drastic the treatment the patient will receive.

There are many ways to prevent breast cancer including Vitamin D, Vitamin E and calcium. Working out four or more hours a week has also proven to help prevent breast cancer. In fact, for some women, exercise decreases the risk of getting breast cancer by as much as 58%. Giving birth before age 20 may also prevent breast cancer. Researchers believe that they can hormonally induce a false pregnancy into a young woman. This will mature the breast tissue and hopefully prevent her from getting breast cancer. High intake of tomatoes may also reduce the risk of breast cancer. If you put your mind to it, you could prevent yourself from getting breast cancer.

Breast cancer is very common in women and yet no cure has been found for it. There are many causes of breast cancer and early detection can and should save lives. Every woman is at risk for getting breast cancer at some point in her life and there are many symptoms. There are many ways to prevent breast cancer and various ways to treat it. Breast cancer should not be fatal. If you or someone you love got diagnosed with breast cancer, what would you do?

END OF GABBY PAPER

DEFINITIONS

Aromatase: The enzyme which makes estrogen out of testosterone and androstenedione.

Aromatase Inhibitors: They stop or block the aromatase enzyme from producing estrogen out of testosterone and androstenedione.

Atypical cells: Abnormal cells.

Atypical hyperplasia: Abnormal cells and too many of the abnormal cells have grown.

Axillary lymph node dissection: The removal of the lymph nodes found under the armpit.

Cytologist: Someone who studies cells.

Excisional biopsy: Removing the entire lump.

Estrogen: A hormone produced by the ovaries, adrenal glands, placenta, and fat. It then circulates through the bloodstream into the breasts and many other areas of the body. Estrogen made by the ovaries decreases gradually during perimenopause and then greatly drops off at menopause.

Hormone therapy: Used as a treatment to decrease or block estrogen thus, decreasing the risk of breast cancer.

In situ: Hasn't left the original site, stays in place.

Incisional biopsy: Removing a part of the lump.

Invasive breast cancer. Has left confines of the original site. May invade the breast tissue, lymph nodes, or other organs in the body.

Metastasis: The spread of cancer to another organ, often through the bloodstream.

Pituitary gland: The head gland in the brain which secretes hormones to regulate other glands.

Premarin: Estrogen from a pregnant horse's urine that is taken after menopause to help alleviate menopausal symptoms.

Progesterone: A hormone produced by the ovaries which is involved in the menstrual cycle.

Sentinel node: The first lymph node under the armpit that the cancer may have gone to.

Sentinel node biopsy. According to the National Cancer Institutes' website a sentinel lymph node biopsy is the "Removal and examination of the sentinel node(s), the first lymph node(s) to which cancer cells are likely to spread from a primary tumor. To identify the sentinel lymph node(s), the surgeon injects a radioactive substance, blue dye, or both near the tumor. The surgeon then uses a scanner to find the sentinel lymph node(s) containing the radioactive substance or looks for the lymph node(s) stained with dye. The surgeon then removes the sentinel node(s) to check for the presence of cancer cells."

Tamoxifen: A drug taken to help tumors sensitive to estrogen =estrogen-receptor-positive tumors.

Disclaimer

Please note that Andrea is not a medical doctor and thus is not intending to give you medical advice. She is merely giving you information that she has gathered and also stating her opinions. Please speak to your doctor with all medical questions and concerns.

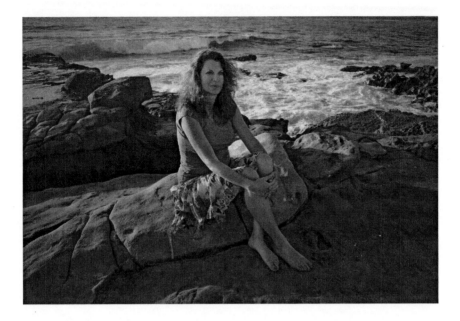

In 2006, at age 41, Andrea learned she had breast cancer. She joined approximately 2.5 million women in the United States who are breast cancer survivors. During her extensive research, the treatment choices offered for early stage breast cancer shocked her. Having her breasts removed as one of the treatment options surprised her the most.

Andrea's skills as an attorney guided her through four years of researching breast cancer and writing this book. She writes from a layperson and survivor's viewpoint rather than from a medical perspective. Andrea lives in San Diego with her two children. She has used her breast cancer experience to transform her personal health and is now in the best physical shape of her life.

Her consultant, Dr. Barry Handler, is a board-certified plastic surgeon with over 10 years of experience in breast reconstruction. His life has been touched personally by the disease, and he takes a special interest in post-mastectomy breast reconstruction. Dr. Handler verified the medical information in this book and contributed vital knowledge for the readers.